To Find
a Way

THE OUTCOME OF
HOSPITAL TREATMENT OF
DISTURBED ADOLESCENTS

To Find a Way

THE OUTCOME OF HOSPITAL TREATMENT OF DISTURBED ADOLESCENTS

John T. Gossett, Ph.D.,
Jerry M. Lewis, M.D.,
and
F. David Barnhart, M.A.

Timberlawn Psychiatric Research Foundation
Dallas, Texas

BRUNNER/MAZEL, *Publishers* • **New York**

Library of Congress Cataloging in Publication Data

Gossett, John T., 1937–
  To find a way.

  Includes index.
  1. Adolescent psychotherapy. 2. Psychiatric
hospital care. I. Lewis, Jerry M., 1924–
II. Barnhart, F. David, 1943–   . III. Title.
[DNLM: 1. Mental disorders—In adolescence.
2. Mental Disorders—Therapy. 3. Hospitals, Psychiatric.
4. Follow-up studies. WS 463 G679t]
RJ503.G67 1983   616.89′14   82-17900
ISBN 0-87630-326-2

Published by
BRUNNER/MAZEL, INC.
19 Union Square
New York, New York 10003

To the Memory of
H. H. F. Gossett

Foreword

The authors of *To Find A Way* have undertaken an ambitious and altruistic task. This task is the sine qua non of hospital treatment evaluation—the long-term outcome follow-up study. Their task is ambitious because in 1966 the authors designed and committed themselves to completing a long-term follow-up of 100 consecutively admitted adolescent inpatients. For 15 years, that commitment has required sustained clinical focus and fund raising. Although the adolescents they followed were severely behavior disordered or schizophrenic, the authors have carried out this task with little attrition. Some of the adolescent patients they have followed now have adolescent children of their own!

The task is altruistic for several reasons. The authors are from the staff of a private psychodynamically oriented hospital and yet they have followed up their *own* hospital's patients with candor and thoroughness, for years and years. Any student of outcome research from such institutions knows that it is far easier to follow-up *other* people's patients. Such a student also knows that to the extent that hospitals like Timberlawn study their own patients, follow-ups are usually self-serving because the emotional investment required by psychotherapists makes a candid contemplation of failure too difficult. Such follow-ups are also usually brief. This is for two reasons. First, most patients seek treatment at clinical nadirs and thus will always improve over the short-term. Second, over the long-term, treatment effects other than one's own become increasingly apparent and that may injure therapeutic vanity. The follow-up by Gossett, Lewis, and Barnhart is neither brief nor self-serving.

To Find A Way is not only ambitious and altruistic; it is also dispassionate and informative. It asks important questions that inpatient treatment staff often ask themselves but despair of answering. On admission, what do patients bring with them that contributes to their long-term outcome? How important is the family matrix? What in the milieu really helps? What treatment interventions work with severely disturbed adolescents and which do not? Are hospital romances good or detrimental to outcome? Will marijuana use after discharge be detrimental? After discharge, how should the emotional impact of a hospitalization that is not of an adolescent's own choosing be dealt with?

In addressing such questions and many others, Gossett, Lewis and Barnhart wisely pay attention to the forest, not the trees. This book neither drowns the authors nor its readers in 16 years' accumulation of minor data. Rather, variables are systematically condensed into global scales; these scales include onset of symptomatology, family evaluation, adolescent psychopathology, and major facets of long-term outcome.

Besides the four virtues to which I have already alluded, common sense, humility, and a sense of perspective are additional qualities that characterize this book. Perhaps the most valuable feature of this book is that it provides collective wisdom from a whole cohort of adolescents who now, grown to maturity, can look back upon what was helpful and what was not helpful about their hospital experience. All those who work with hospitalized psychiatric patients will learn from *To Find A Way.*

George E. Vaillant, M.D.

Contents

APPENDICES

Preface

The Timberlawn Adolescent Treatment Assessment Project was designed to provide treatment outcome information useful to mental health professionals. Material from the project is organized in three sections. The first provides background information describing our initial interest in treatment assessment; the second section details results of the project. Clinical and research implications are discussed in the third section. The following resumé of chapters indicates the flow of this material.

Chapter 1 presents clinical vignettes to highlight the typical issues of planning treatment that demonstrate the need for detailed long-term outcome assessment. Clinical and research problems involved in the planning and conduct of the study are presented.

Chapter 2 provides a comprehensive review of published follow-up studies and integrates prognostic and treatment planning findings emerging from the review. Adolescent follow-up studies are organized by patient, family, and treatment variables. Adult hospital follow-up studies are summarized as well.

Chapter 3 describes the clinical findings relevant to prognosis and treatment planning of three pilot studies involving 56 patients. Information on the hospital setting, the sample of patients, the treatment program, initial follow-up procedures, and early measurement techniques are detailed.

Chapter 4 explains the development of the research design resulting from the pilot studies. These methodological developments and data depicting the levels of function at follow-up for 120 patients in the Main Study are presented.

Chapter 5 focuses an analysis in depth of the patients, their response to the treatment program, and the course of their lives several years beyond the hospital treatment experience. Data gathered at the time of hospital admission, throughout the course of the treatment program, and during the period from discharge to follow-up are assessed for their relationships to long-term levels of function.

Chapter 6 details measurement techniques that reflect several important clinical dimensions: severity and chronicity of psychopathology, family level of competence, and locus of control. The relationships of scores on these clinical scales to eventual outcome are presented.

Chapter 7 presents material along two dimensions of the treatment program. First, the relationships of patterns of medication usage to eventual outcome are examined. Second, measures of patients' relationships with each other and with staff are explored for their prognostic and treatment planning utility.

Chapter 8 describes the evaluation of a model of multivariate predictions of outcome.

Chapter 9 explores a variety of patient, family, staff, and program issues at a clinical level.

Chapter 10 summarizes a rationale for hospital evaluation studies and suggests an optimal organization of such studies and the resolution of problems and conflicts frequently encountered.

OVERVIEW

This project required substantial expenditure of time, effort, and financial resources. It seems relevant at this point to provide an outline overview of findings of the project that we believe justify follow-up treatment assessment study.

1) The most important finding of the study is that treatment outcome was successful for approximately two-thirds of the 176 patients, despite the unusual severity and chronicity of their presenting problems. In an era of widespread skepticism concerning the efficacy of psychiatric treatment in general and the need for long-term hospitali-

zation of selected patients in particular, this finding is of considerable professional and social importance.

2) Results from this study, combined with those of previous studies, highlight the importance to prognosis and treatment planning of the assessment of severity and chronicity of patients' psychopathology, intelligence, family level of competence, locus of control, interpersonal relationships, and continuing psychotherapy following discharge. Additionally, hospital factors of basic importance include providing a specialized adolescent treatment program; completing inpatient goals; developing innovative treatment approaches for certain patient groups; using relatively small, semi-autonomous, decision-sharing treatment units with high staff-patient ratios; and planning discharge and transitional care facilities.

3) The importance of continuing to improve methods of measuring patient, family, staff, and program variables is emphasized.

4) In order to achieve multivariate data analysis accurately reflecting clinical complexities, it is crucial to have a variety of proven measurement techniques in place at the beginning of follow-up study.

5) Results from this study offer tentative guidelines for an optimal matching of treatment programs to patient and family problems and needs. This information is a step in planning empirically grounded, individualized treatment.

6) The variety of patient, family, staff, and program findings, obtained several years after discharge, contains meaningful implications for optimal hospital treatment planning and management.

7) Numerous issues involved in the integration of follow-up treatment assessment into an ongoing clinical program are described, along with suggestions for their resolution. It is hoped that this material will stimulate follow-up treatment assessment in other psychiatric hospitals.

Acknowledgments

The Timberlawn Adolescent Treatment Assessment Project involved the combined efforts of many individuals over an extended period of time. Without the cooperation of clinical personnel, the project could not have been accomplished. All staff members of the Adolescent Service participated in data collection, and their ongoing critique and enthusiastic involvement kept the project alive. In addition to key support from the nursing supervisors, the assistance of three psychiatrists was crucial. We owe special thanks to Joe W. King, M.D., Doyle I. Carson, M.D., and Roy H. Fanoni, M.D.

A number of research personnel made important contributions to the project. Susan B. Lewis, M.A., a research sociologist, played a vital role in project design and data collection in the early years. Virginia Austin Phillips, the Foundation's Senior Research Associate, provided valuable assistance throughout the project. This ranged from initial design and data collection through final editing of the manuscript. The bulk of the never-ceasing secretarial work was contributed by Norma Muldoon, Nannette Bruchey, Virginia Zinchak, and Deborah Haubrich, and we are grateful for both their expertise and patience.

We wish to thank the editors of the following publications for their permission to reprint portions of material published earlier: *American*

Journal of Orthopsychiatry, Archives of General Psychiatry, Adolescence, Southern Medical Journal, Journal of the National Association of Private Psychiatric Hospitals, Jason Aronson, Inc., and Sage Publications, Inc.

Funding longitudinal research is a never-ending problem. All of the support for this research came from private sources—foundations and interested individuals. During the early years, the birth of the project was made possible by a grant from The Hoblitzelle Foundation. Survival of the project was insured by subsequent support from The Charles B. Goddard Foundation, The Florence Foundation, The Samuel Roberts Noble Foundation, Inc., the Crystal Charity Ball, and the Timberlawn Psychiatric Hospital. A large number of individuals played major roles both in obtaining grants and in providing leadership to the Board of the Timberlawn Psychiatric Research Foundation. R. Vernon Coe, Leo Patterson, Jr., James M. Moroney, Jr., David L. Florence, and James W. Aston played crucial roles. Through all the uncertainties of funding for psychiatric research, Charles and Sarah Seay have been the people we could turn to for whatever was necessary. They always came through and, more than anyone else, are responsible for this and our other projects.

The cooperation of the patients and families who comprise this study was, of course, essential. Despite their pain they participated—often only because the project held some hope for diminishing someone else's pain in the future. We are grateful for their courage.

Finally, our wives, Karen, Pat, and Reid, tolerated our frequent preoccupation and were open in support of the project. For this and much more we are thankful.

JOHN T. GOSSETT, Ph.D.
JERRY M. LEWIS, M.D.
F. DAVID BARNHART, M.A.

Upon this gifted age, in its dark hour,
Rains from the sky a meteoric shower
Of facts . . . they lie unquestioned, uncombined.
Wisdom enough to leech us of our ill
Is daily spun; but there exists no loom
To weave it into fabric. . . .

Edna St. Vincent Millay

To Find
a Way

THE OUTCOME OF
HOSPITAL TREATMENT OF
DISTURBED ADOLESCENTS

PART I

Background

CHAPTER 1

Introduction

A young woman recalls her first encounter with a psychiatric hospital.

Interviewer: Think back to the time you were admitted to the hospital, and tell me what was going on with you back then.

Jane: Okay, I think that I had sort of lost time; time didn't have anything to do with anything else, including day and night. I think for several weeks before I came I spent a lot of time in bed staring at the ceiling because I really couldn't do much of anything else. Before that, before I had been put on medication, I was out of control. I was scared and it seemed like I had set things in motion, but I didn't know where they were going, and in some ways maybe it was a conscious moving toward a climax, but not having any idea what it would be like. Things couldn't continue the way they were, and I guess I would have been as crazy as I needed to be to get out of the situation I was in.

It was terrible at home. Everybody was fighting. Physically fighting. I was afraid. I was afraid we were going to kill each other. I had no control over what I was doing in school; I think that control was really a big issue. I didn't seem to be able to change or equalize anything. It was like being on a rollercoaster, but it didn't stop on the first round or the second round—it just kept going and going. I was having terrible nightmares when I slept, nightmares that someone would be killed. Somebody was going to go crazy and kill everybody. I remember one nightmare: When I came in the house, there was blood all over. I never actually saw any bodies, but there was just blood everywhere. That may have been when I started cutting myself—I'm not sure. But I had a feeling a lot of times that there was a part of me that was somewhere above it all watching it happen and wondering if I was doing this . . . if I was really doing this . . . if maybe I was in control of it after all, and not being able to find out— not being able to figure it out.

I had been seeing Dr. Allen, and I remember the first time I saw him he said to me, "Have you considered hospitalization?" I guess he thought I was pretty crazy, but I'm not sure. I had put myself in the company of a lot of crazy kids; some had been here, and it was sort of like maybe it would work if I was in the hospital. I think that most of the negotiation was done with my knowledge—not all of it, but a lot of it. Everybody in the family was real upset about the possibility of hospitalization, and we all kept changing our minds, back and forth. It was so scary.

I hadn't been able to do anything in school for a long time. My friend could come and pick me up from one class and deposit me in my next class, and I just sat there. I would fall asleep in class, you know, because of the medication. I am sure it really scared my teachers.

The day I came—I can even remember what I wore. I had on a corduroy suit. I was afraid that my parents would change their minds. I remember we came in the two-door car, and that was very unusual because that's not the car we usually drove. I guess that I had convinced them that I didn't really want to be here to please them—and I suppose they were afraid that I might jump out of the car.

I remember it was like being drunk and riding in a car and just being carried along, and it didn't really matter where you were going or what was happening. It was a long drive, with lots of curves and ups and downs, and then all of a sudden we were here. It was really strange. There was still the possibility they wouldn't leave me because I was acting like I didn't want to be here. My parents were scared to death, and so was I. The doctor asked me some questions, and I barely answered them because I didn't really know what to do.

When I said goodbye to my parents, it was a very peculiar, flat unemotional experience, like I was watching from somewhere else. And then somebody took me over to the Unit, and they opened the door, and I went in, and it closed behind me, and I heard it lock. It made a *big* noise when it closed and locked. Once I was here, I just sat and stared into space, I think. People would come up and ask me questions, but I was so scared I just sat and stared. Some of the people frightened me. I guess I was pretty scary to them, too.

This successful 30-year-old woman describes very clearly the complicated fears and hopes she experienced when she was admitted to a psychiatric hospital as an adolescent. She can describe with equal clarity many events during the ensuing months that were experienced as very helpful and a number that were experienced as decidedly unhelpful. Most of this material, however, was unavailable to the doctors and others working with Jane* during her hospitalization. In part, this was because she was unable at that time to be as clear in her descriptions, but in part, it was also because her fear, ambivalence, and desperate self-protection were often viewed by the staff as stubborn oppositionalism—an interpretation not conducive to sharing.

During the course of working with Jane, staff would have found it very difficult to predict her long-term outcome with any degree of specificity. What was much more troubling to staff at that time was a series of questions: Are we helping? How are we helping? How should we best deal with her parents? How should we organize the overall treatment experience to give her the best chance to function adaptively in the future? Which aspects of her behavior in the hospital predict how she will act after she leaves?

At the inception of this project in 1966, two of the authors (JTG, JML) were involved in organizing an inpatient adolescent service, and there were few empirical guidelines to suggest that any one treatment approach was superior to any other. Obvious, however, was the ex-

---

*A pseudonym.

treme severity and chronicity of personal and family difficulties encountered by patients referred for intermediate- to long-term treatment because they had not progressed satisfactorily in outpatient or
prior short-term inpatient treatment. We knew that over the course of
our work we would have both successes and failures, and we hoped to
establish reliable information that would help us improve the treatment program. Although there was little evidence available at that
time, it was possible that treatment response within the hospital would
not necessarily predict long-term outcome. Thus was born our commitment to collect data on patients, their families, and certain aspects
of the treatment experience for correlation later with long-term, posthospital functioning.

Our first patients are now in their thirties; some have adolescent
children of their own. Many keep in touch, to tell us how their lives are
going or to ask for assistance from time to time. These occasions teach
us more about the strengths and shortcomings of the treatment program.

Many problems are encountered during the conduct of a follow-up
study. Which aspects of the patient, family, and treatment program
should be measured during hospitalization? Scores of ideas need to be
considered. Each colleague who is consulted has different ideas concerning the "crucial" variables that must be assessed out of the hun-
dreds that could be measured. How is one to choose?

Who will measure and record the data? Clinicians in a hospital setting have little "spare time." If research personnel are to be hired, can
funding be obtained?

Will ongoing research designed to assess the quality of care interfere
with clinical practice? Treatment outcome research is easy to favor,
but often proves to be stressful to practicing clinicians because it is difficult to separate the outcome of treatment from their own assets and
liabilities. Will research needs interfere with clinical decisions? Research personnel need to have enough power in a treatment system to
accomplish their work; will this interfere with optimal treatment?

Since some follow-up work from other hospitals has already been
published, is there any point in conducting another study? In order to
provide a genuine contribution to clinical practice, a study must offer
something over and above prior studies—but what?

What will be the implications if one finds that few patients have been helped?

Can highly mobile former patients be located several years after discharge? If we are not able to locate almost all the former patients, will results be sufficiently biased to be of little, if any, value? If former patients and their parents are located, will they be cooperative in a venture that offers a great deal to the researchers but very little to them?

Can former patients' accounts of their personal successes and failures be trusted? Are advisers correct who suggest that the combination of unconscious defenses and conscious deceptions render their accounts useless for the assessment of treatment? When the former patients live apart from their parents at the time of follow-up, are parents' observations valid?

Will a lengthy follow-up interview stimulate regression in vulnerable individuals? Are the gains from follow-up interviews worth the risk of being harmful to former patients whose adaptations may be tenuous at the time of follow-up contact?

If follow-up information can be obtained, how will one assess the level of outcome? As some suggest, is rate of rehospitalization the best measure of long-term outcome? Or, at the other extreme, do subtle, intrapsychic processes need assessment? Or are scales for a variety of overt behaviors better? What are the criteria for selecting one means of measuring life effectiveness instead of others?

What method of gathering follow-up information is to be used: questionnaires, telephone contacts, personal interviews, or psychological tests? What are the practical consequences of each approach?

Assuming that an adequate number of former patients demonstrating effective life functioning were found, how can "treatment success" be distinguished from "spontaneous remission"? Might those who achieve effective levels of life functioning have done as well without lengthy, expensive, and often painful inpatient treatment?

Is it preferable to have treatment staff do the follow-up interview, or clinically skilled persons with no previous contact with the former patients? Can former treatment staff be objective in assessing the long-term outcome of persons they have treated? From the opposite point of view, can interviewers who do not know the former patients or their parents elicit their cooperation?

Finally, after obtaining information both during the course of hospitalization and at the time of outcome, how can the intricate relationships between patient, family, and treatment variables and subsequent level of functioning be clarified? When all patients and families are involved in a "total push" milieu program involving a host of complex treatment variables, how can one determine what really helps, what is irrelevant, and what has failed to help, or what has been harmful?

This research project sought answers to these and other complex questions.

In intensive hospital treatment programs, clinicians must endure discomfort, frustration, and uncertainty. Failures are all too obvious; successes are often difficult to understand. Successes, however, do occur, and we are getting better at understanding them.

Many years after her hospitalization, Jane wrote:

I remember watching the changing of time
　　from the antiseptic inside of a locked cage
　　with glass windows.
I remember every fiber of my mind and body
　　straining against captivity
　　screaming to be set free
To feel the air—to smell the storms
　　that mean spring.
To run in the rain
　　and roll in the grass
To talk to the squirrels
　　and just to cry—
　　alone.
And I remember the day
　　when I realized
That to want all these things
　　was the will to live.
From that day
　　I am alive
And I never said thank you
　　and
I never said I love you.

This poem expresses a gratitude rarely received during the course of treatment by those involved in providing it. While the gratitude and affection are warming, the transcendent rewards include the knowledge that one participated in saving her life, in helping others, and in trying to learn more about how to be helpful.

Another vignette may emphasize the dual purposes of this research.

Jason B.,* a 15-year-old male, was transferred from the psychiatric unit of a local general hospital where he had been for nine weeks. The referring psychiatrist indicated that he was unmanageable on that unit; he had attacked a nurse, led a riot, set two fires, and consistently disrupted unit activities.

Jason's psychiatric history was lengthy and complex. His parents described him as a difficult baby, hard to hold, and with severe colic. As a preschool child he was intensely "independent" and, unlike his older siblings, seemed little interested in family activities. From the beginning of school he had been a problem for his teachers. His academic performance had been poor, although repeated testing indicated normal intelligence. Because of his disruptive behavior he was expelled from four schools.

At age nine he was seen in a child guidance clinic, but he refused to cooperate with the recommended outpatient psychotherapy. When he was 11, a child psychiatrist recommended placing him in a residential school, but his parents declined. At 13 he was incarcerated briefly in a junvenile detention center following his arrest for breaking a plate glass window in a neighborhood store. At 14 he was briefly hospitalized in the psychiatric unit of a local general hospital when he threatened his parents with a knife. An attempt to involve him in outpatient psychotherapy following hospitalization failed, and three months later he was admitted again to that unit for "increasing unmanageability" at home.

Jason was the youngest of three male children. His oldest brother was described as studious, hard-working, and an "excellent, if somewhat quiet, boy." The second son, a senior in high

---

*Identities have been disguised to protect confidentiality.

school, was an average student and an outstanding football
player. The parents, both in their early forties, indicated that they
had a "good" marriage and, with the exception of the problems
with Jason, a "strong" family. Jason's father, a successful attor-
ney, was heavily involved in politics and civic affairs. His mother,
the daughter of a prominent family, was active in many charitable
organizations. The parents appeared to be overwhelmed by
Jason's behavior and their inability to arrange for successful
treatment. They acknowledged openly their opinion that there
was something basically wrong with Jason which they thought
was "chemical." There was no family history of mental illness.

During the initial weeks of hospitalization, Jason defied the
staff and, despite staff efforts and intense confrontation by fellow patients in the daily unit meetings, his aggressive behavior es-
calated, resulting in several periods of physical restraint. During
his third week of hospitalization the therapist's observations,
along with the unit staff observations, psychological testing, family assessment, and physical and neurological studies resulted in
the initial clinical formulation. Jason was seen as having a severe
personality disorder, with borderline personality organization
and increasing antisocial tendencies; developmental psychopathology centering about the separation-individuation period with
associated primitive defenses; a predominant underlying empty,
depressive affect, a frightened avoidance of all intimacy, and intense rage. Despite the family's surface appearance, results of the
formal family assessment indicated severe, chronic family dysfunction. Jason's parents' relationship was clearly dominant-submissive with the father rigidly controlling the mother. In turn,
Jason's mother was quietly angry, and there was evidence of her
vicarious enjoyment when the father was unable to control
Jason's behavior.

Jason was hospitalized for 17 months. After four months of intense resistance, he began to participate in a variety of therapeutic
activities: He became intensely involved with his individual therapist, gradually came to be a working member of his psychotherapy group and, after a year of hospitalization, became a leader in
the protreatment group process on his unit. His work in the hospi-

tal school gradually became task-oriented, and he developed an important relationship with a teacher. He also developed a close relationship with the evening nurse on his unit and often spent time talking with her late at night. His parents were seen in marital therapy and made some progress in reorienting their relationship. During the latter months of Jason's hospitalization, family therapy was started. Although Jason's hospital course was tumultuous in the early months, it later developed a relatively smooth pattern of effective and multiple therapeutic involvements.

At the time of discharge, Jason was described as "markedly improved." His use of splitting, projection, and a variety of interpersonal distancing maneuvers had disappeared. His relationship with a patient on the girls' unit showed some evidence of closeness and emotional intimacy. Discharge plans involved his return to the family home, reentry into public school, and continuation of individual, group, and family therapy.

At the time of follow-up, Jason was 21 years old and lived in an apartment with his girlfriend. He attended a community college part time and worked at a filling station owned by a family friend. His parents assisted him economically. He had not been in any legal difficulty. His plans for the future were hazy but centered about automobiles—"fixing them, owning them, racing them." He had continued individual psychotherapy for two years, group psychotherapy for six months, and family therapy for one year. He continued to have occasional contacts with his individual therapist, most often at times of stress such as breaking up with a girlfriend. He felt "pretty good" about himself "most of the time." His parents were pleased with his treatment although candid about their opinion that he would not achieve as his older brothers were. "He's got a good chance now," his father said, "and his mother and I are much, much better."

This vignette reflects the difficult kind of clinical work that underlies this book. On the surface, evaluation of treatment outcome in this instance seems reasonably clear. A mid-adolescent boy who seemed headed for a life of trouble appears to be "making it." The clinical material, however, raises as many questions as it answers. One of these is the need to understand what combination of factors—patient, family, and treatment—in concert account for the apparent success of a massive, difficult, time-consuming, and expensive intervention. The answer is of particular significance when one considers that the clinical vignette might have focused on another patient, who, on the surface, would not appear much different, but for whom the intervention failed and at follow-up was found to be making only a marginal community adjustment, hospitalized, imprisoned, or dead.

In order to answer such a question, this book weaves together two themes: first, the treatment of disturbed adolescents in a psychiatric hospital and the outcome of that treatment; second, the importance of treatment evaluation follow-up studies.

CHAPTER 2

The Evaluation of Psychiatric Hospital Treatment

Intensive inpatient psychiatric care for adolescents has been available in this country for approximately 60 years.[6] Although clinicians recognized the crucial significance of long-term follow-up assessment of treatment, translations of that realization into published reports have been rare. The small number of informal follow-up studies before 1958 focused almost exclusively upon adolescent schizophrenic patients, despite clinical reports demonstrating that many adolescents treated in psychiatric hospitals had affective psychoses, disabling neuroses, organically-determined behavioral disorders, or antisocial or aggressive behavior problems.[7,8,15,27]

The first detailed account of a long-term follow-up assessment of a representative sample of adolescent inpatients was published by Masterson in 1958.[26] This chapter will review 22 adolescent follow-up studies located in a comprehensive literature search and summarize and integrate material reviewing adult inpatient follow-up research.

The four criteria used exclude a number of follow-up reports only peripherally related to our major interests: 1) The treatment services must have been of an inpatient nature; 2) the subjects must have been hospitalized during adolescence (approximately ages 13–19); 3) the interval between hospital discharge and follow-up must have been at least six months; and 4) the study must have included correlations of patient, family, or treatment variables with the patient's level of function at the time of follow-up.

Methodology varies widely in the studies. Generally researchers did not replicate previous work, and thus reports are not readily comparable. The studies, for example, emanate from different hospitals with treatment programs for patients with demographic, diagnostic, and behavioral differences. Criteria for measurement of change also vary from study to study, yet there are significant commonalities. All examine adolescents or young adults at least six months after discharge from inpatient facilities. All subjects were inpatients during some part of their adolescence, and most were young adults at the time of follow-up. The most common diagnoses were severe personality disorder and psychosis. Each study includes judgments of patient change, either in terms of improvement (change from admission to time of follow-up), level of function (status relative to "normality"), or both. In each study, relationships between patient, family, or treatment variables and treatment outcome are explored.

This chapter focuses upon seven variables found in several studies to be related significantly to long-term outcome. Three of these variables concern the patients themselves (severity of psychopathology, process versus reactive onset of symptomatology, and intelligence). One variable is that of the patient's family's level of function. Two correlates refer to the nature of the hospital treatment (presence of a specialized adolescent program and the completion of hospital treatment). One factor pertains to aftercare (continuation of psychotherapy following hospital discharge). Selected material from adult follow-up studies is included, and these findings are integrated with the results from the follow-up studies of adolescent patients.

PATIENT VARIABLES

Severity of Patient Psychopathology

Clearly the most powerful prognostic sign at the time of a teenager's admission to a psychiatric hospital is an evaluation of severity of psychopathology. The level of function at follow-up relates inversely to this initial measure; that is, the less the initial disturbance, the better the level of function at follow-up. Fifteen of the 22 investigators report severity of psychopathology, with the most typical measure that of diagnostic level; that is, neurosis, personality disorder, or psychosis.[1,2,4,12,14,16-19,23,24,26,28,34,35] All studies reviewed were published prior to adoption of DSM-III and, accordingly, patients referred to as "neurotic" generally display severely phobic and/or depressive symptomatology in the absence of psychotic symptoms or those suggesting a profound personality disorder. Using DSM-III criteria, most such patients would receive an Axis I diagnosis of anxiety or dysthymic disorder, and an Axis II diagnosis of histrionic, dependent, or compulsive personality disorder. Patients referred to as "personality disorders" are primarily those who currently would receive a severe personality disorder diagnosis and reflect a predominance of acting-out behaviors. The majority of patients described in these studies as "psychotic" would currently receive a primary diagnosis of either a schizophrenic or major affective disorder.

Although the average level of severity of disturbance differs between neurosis, personality disorder, and psychosis, there is some overlap. Differences in criteria of severity of disturbance and levels of function at follow-up make strict comparisons open to question. However, 80–90 percent of those inpatients diagnosed as neurotic are functioning reasonably well at follow-up. A smaller proportion, perhaps between one-quarter and one-third, of those diagnosed as psychotic are significantly improved or functioning well at follow-up. Adolescent patients with a personality disorder diagnosis show a wide range of long-term function from study to study, with an average success rate of between 50 and 60 percent.

Process Versus Reactive Onset of Symptomatology

A number of studies of adult schizophrenic patients find that illnesses diagnosed "reactive" have a better prognosis than those diagnosed "process."[13,20-22] For many years the distinction between process and reactive has been applied solely to schizophrenic disorders; more recently the concept has been generalized to apply as well to other types of psychiatric disorders.[13,36,37] While application of the process-reactive continuum to other forms of psychopathology may be unfamiliar to some clinicians, there are both theoretical and empirical reasons to support its usefulness (see Chapter 3). The characteristics used to define process and reactive types of disturbances are summarized in Table 1; findings relating these characteristics to outcome with adolescent patients are reviewed below.

TABLE 1

Criteria for Differentiating Process and Reactive Psychopathology*

Process Disorder	Reactive Disorder
Birth to 5th Year	
1. Severe psychological trauma	1. No severe psychological trauma
2. Frequent or severe physical illness	2. Good physical health
3. Patient considered "odd" child in the family	3. Patient considered "normal" child in the family
5th Year to Adolescence	
4. Academic failures	4. Academic success
5. Introversion; isolation from peers	5. Extroversion; involvement with peers
6. Disturbed siblings	6. Normal siblings
Adolescence to Adulthood	
7. Marked verbal and physical passivity	7. Verbally and physically active; normal assertiveness
8. Absence of heterosexual behavior	8. Presence of heterosexual behavior
9. Gradual onset of disabling symptoms	9. Sudden onset of disabling symptoms
10. Lack of clear stress precipitating symptoms	10. Clear stress precipitating symptoms
11. Early onset of severe psychopathology	11. Late onset of severe psychopathology
12. Bland, insidious onset of symptoms	12. Intense, "stormy" onset of symptoms
13. Slow symptomatic response to hospitalization	13. Rapid symptomatic improvement with hospitalization

*Adapted from Garmezy[13] and Kantor and Herron.[22]

Early Psychological Trauma

The strongest preadmission predictor of outcome in the study by Masterson and Costello[28] is a measure of "Life Stress" which includes estimates of the impact of highly disruptive events occurring in the patient's early life. Other studies, however, do not find this variable useful in predicting outcome.[19]

Childhood Physical Illness

The single follow-up study that explores the relationship between early childhood physical illness and later psychiatric outcome produces no significant association.[34]

Evidence of "Oddness" in Early Childhood

The investigation perhaps most nearly relevant to this dimension was conducted by Masterson.[26] He states that the presence of "neuropathic" traits (tantrums, feeding problems, breath holding, enuresis, night terrors, ticks, and nail biting) in the early life of schizophrenic patients is not predictive of eventual outcome.

Academic Failures

Masterson[27] reports that schizophrenics and those with personality disorders who pass all grades up to the time of hospitalization have better outcomes than those who have failed one or more subjects or grades. Pollack et al.[30] also find that grade failure or remedial help in the academic experiences of adolescent patients is predictive of poor outcome. They specifically link evidence of early academic failure with the process-reactive dimension. Two other studies report similar results.[5,16]

Isolation from Peers

Results from six studies tend to support peer relationships in early childhood as a predictor of long-term outcome. Carter[8] finds that psychotic children who have early shown " . . . defects in amiability, shyness, sensitiveness, loneliness, and moodiness. . ." tend to have poor outcome, whereas those with a history of amiability and warmth of personality tend to have good outcome. Masterson[26] finds that ability to relate both to individuals and to groups predicts positive outcome for his schizophrenic patients, but this does not hold true for neurotic or personality disorder individuals. Pollack et al.[30] and Masterson and Costello[28] find that friendships both before and during adolescence are predictors of positive outcome, while Hartmann et al.[19] and Grob and Singer[16] find similar results for friendships during adolescence. In the latter four studies, psychotic and personality disorder patients are combined.

Disturbed Siblings

No studies specifically relating evaluation of adolescent patients at follow-up to the presence of disturbed siblings were found.

Marked Passivity

The study of Hartmann et al.[19] demonstrates that patients with a history of marked inhibition of aggressive affect have poor outcome. Carter[8] and Pollack et al.[30] also find that patients described as shy, shut-in, passive, or withdrawn have a poorer prognosis than do those showing average or above-average levels of activity or aggressiveness.

Heterosexual Behavior

Neither the study of Hartmann et al.[19] nor that of Pollack et al.[30] finds the presence or absence of heterosexual behavior in the past history of adolescent patients to be helpful in predicting outcome.

Gradual Onset of Symptoms

Carter,[8] Hartmann et al.,[19] and Masterson[26] find gradual onset to be predictive of poor outcome, while acute onset is related to a more positive treatment result.

Precipitating Events

Three studies deal with the influence of precipitating factors. Carter[8] finds that with schizophrenic adolescents it is rarely possible to identify factors precipitating the psychotic disorder and that, even when they can be identified, they lack predictive significance. For non-schizophrenic patients, however, the presence of clear precipitating factors predicts better prognosis. The predictive significance of the presence of a precipitating factor was supported in the one-year (but not the 10-year) assessment for the Hartmann et al.[19] sample, but not by Masterson.[26] Thus, the significance of a precipitating factor as a predictor appears equivocal.

Age of Onset

The recovery rate in Carter's[8] sample of psychotic adolescents in whom the onset of illness occurred before age 17 is only 10 percent. When the onset occurs later, the recovery rate is 55 percent. In Masterson's[27] sample of schizophrenic patients, those admitted after the age of 15 have a better recovery rate than do those who are hospitalized at younger ages. The opposite, however, is true of Masterson's[26] patients diagnosed as personality disorders; that is, the younger the patient at admission, the better the prognosis. Warren[34] finds that psychotic patients with early onset have poor outcome; this is not true, however, in his group of teenagers with either neurotic or personality disorders. Teenagers in the study by Hartmann et al.[19] who experience disabling symptoms before age 12½ initially have poor outcomes, but this finding does not hold at 10 years. Schizophrenic patients in another study also show a significant relationship between age of first psychiatric contact and outcome.[30] Those with the best outcome are those who are oldest at first treatment contact. Aarkrog et al.,[1] following a group of teenagers with a variety of diagnoses, find that early onset of illness is a bad prognostic sign, as do Grob and Singer.[16]

It is clear that in psychosis the earlier the age of onset (particularly if prepubertal), the poorer the prognosis. In neurosis or personality disorder, however, the relationship of age of onset is equivocal.

Intensity of Onset

In Carter's[8] psychotic group, the more stormy the onset, the better the prognosis. In Masterson's[27] schizophrenic sample, those showing an onset characterized by confusion or fear tend to have a better outcome than do those showing autism or shallow affect.

Rate of Symptomatic Improvement with Hospitalization

A final process-reactive factor is the rate of symptomatic improvement occurring during early nonspecific treatment in the hospital milieu. In Carter's[8] sample of psychotic adolescents, most who recover show marked symptom clearance during the first three months of hospitalization. Masterson's[26] schizophrenics and personality disorders have a much higher rate of recovery if they demonstrate rapid symptomatic improvement soon after hospitalization. This variable does not predict outcome, however, with neurotic patients.

In summary, when evaluating psychotic adolescents, a configuration of seven factors suggests a process disorder with poor prognosis: a history of academic failure; isolation from peers; extreme passivity; early, gradual, and bland onset of symptoms; and a slow symptomatic response to the nonspecific aspects of hospital treatment. For those patients diagnosed neurotic or personality disorder, the process-reactive dimension seems a less powerful predictor. However, a similar configuration of factors also appears related to negative outcome.

Intelligence

Findings from seven studies suggest that below-average intelligence (tested intelligent quotients of less than 90) is correlated with poor long-term outcome.[2,5,8,19,25,30,34]

FAMILY VARIABLES

Early investigators exploring family backgrounds for a history of psychosis, severe alcoholism, or family separations report no significant relationship between such items in the family history and the patient's subsequent long-term function.[2,19,26] These results are similar to longitudinal studies comparing disturbed and well-functioning non-hospitalized teenagers which reveal no significant differences based on the simple presence or absence of family psychosis or marked trauma.[9,29,31-33] These comparison studies do reveal significant differences, however, between normal and abnormal teenagers in coping skills learned in the family setting. This finding suggests that more subtle measures of family dysfunction might be predictive.

In exploring overall severity of family psychopathology, Carter[8] notes that a family history with a single occurrence of psychosis, delinquency, epilepsy, alcoholism, neurosis, or personality disorder does not predict outcome. However, in cases with *multiple* signs of family disturbance, treatment outcome is almost invariably poor:

> As regards the group of non-recovery cases, 17 out of 47 showed abnormality in the parents. This is 36 percent compared with 17 percent in the fully recovered. There is also a difference in the quality of the abnormality, the parents either being more obviously psychotic or more eccentric and introverted. . . .[8]

This finding also suggests that the level of family dysfunction (rather than the presence of particular, circumscribed, individual diagnostic descriptors) might be more sensitive in predicting treatment outcome. Studies relying upon more sensitive means of detecting family level of dysfunction find significant relationships between severity of family dysfunction and the eventual adult functioning of the individual patient.[1,5,16,17,28]

TREATMENT VARIABLES

Treatment variables have been examined less frequently than patient variables, but attempts to correlate various aspects of treatment programs with long-term outcome produce three factors that are clearly significant: a hospital program oriented specifically toward adolescents rather than incorporating them into adult programs; the degree to which patients complete the recommended inpatient treatment; and continuation of psychotherapy after discharge.

Special Adolescent Programs

Data compiled by Beavers and Blumberg[4] suggest that hospitals offering a specialized adolescent treatment program have better long-term results, especially for schizophrenic and personality disorder patients. This observation is supported in other studies.[5,12,14,23,25,30]

Although it is difficult to compare all aspects of the specialized adolescent treatment approaches being described by the various investigators, one common feature is the presence of an educational program for the hospitalized patients.

Completion of Inpatient Treatment

In Levy's[25] study, 85 percent of the teenagers who complete the recommended inpatient treatment have a successful long-term outcome. In contrast, among patients whose hospital treatment is terminated by the institution, only 33 percent have a successful outcome. The institution terminates treatment if there are highly limiting organic factors, institutional inability to manage the patient, or need for a different type of treatment facility. When a patient's parents terminate treatment because they decide the patient does not need treatment or are dissatisfied, discouraged, or angry at the hospital, 58 percent have a successful long-term course. Although failure to complete treatment may be a reflection of the severity of family and patient psychopathology rather than an independent variable, similar results are obtained in three other studies.[1,14,16]

Continuation of Psychotherapy

For most teenagers who receive intensive inpatient treatment, the period of hospitalization is but the first phase of a planned, long-range treatment program. Extended individual, group, and family psychotherapy frequently are recommended at the time of hospital discharge. Some patients and their families accept the recommendations for such aftercare, but others do not.

Hartmann et al.[19] find that continuing psychotherapy after discharge leads to better long-term outcome. Beavers and Blumberg[4] report that 80 percent of those who continue psychotherapy and 41 percent of those who discontinue are significantly improved at follow-up. Similar results appear in three additional studies.[14,16,28] Continuation of psychotherapy after discharge may be an indirect measure of severity of psychopathology; that is, generally healthier patients and their family members are more apt to continue.

Those variables found to have insignificant, contradictory, or undetermined relationships to long-term outcome are summarized in Table 2.

SUMMARY OF ADOLESCENT STUDIES

From 22 long-term follow-up studies of the inpatient psychiatric treatment of adolescents published between 1942 and 1980, seven factors correlate at statistically significant levels with long-range outcome: 1) severity of patient psychopathology; 2) process versus reactive onset of symptomatology; 3) intelligence; 4) severity of family dysfunction; 5) a specialized adolescent treatment program; 6) completion of the recommended hospital treatment; and 7) continuation of recommended psychotherapy after hospitalization. The establishment of these factors should encourage the testing of other variables, despite the number of measures that fail to correlate with treatment outcome at their present level of sensitivity (Table 2).

SUMMARY OF ADULT STUDIES

In contrast to the small number of follow-up studies of adolescents treated in psychiatric hospitals, there are many detailing the outcome of psychiatric hospital treatment of adults. The results of these studies are summarized in two exhaustive review articles.[3,11] It is fortunate that, while follow-up studies of adolescents focus on patient characteristics that influence long-term outcome, adult hospital follow-up studies more often focus upon treatment or hospital system correlates of patients' outcome status, thus providing needed balance.

Anthony et al.[3] rely upon recidivism and employment as primary outcome criteria; they indicate that a preponderance of adult studies yield average rates of rehospitalization of 40 to 50 percent one year after discharge, and 20 to 30 percent have full-time employment at the same follow-up interval. They review a variety of treatment innovations against these "baseline" data obtained from "traditional" treatment programs and report four basic findings:

1) Almost any type of inpatient treatment innovation improves behavior of patients during hospitalization.

TABLE 2

Variables with Statistically Non-significant, Contradictory, or Undetermined Relationship to Long-term Level of Function

Prehospital Variables

1. Age at hospital admission
2. Attitudes towards idealism, rebellion, and religion
3. Birth order
4. Diagnostic subtypes, or patterns of symptoms
5. EEG results
6. Family moves
7. Family psychosis
8. Grandparents in the home
9. Legal difficulties
10. Physical maturity
11. Previous drug therapy
12. Previous psychiatric hospitalization
13. Religion
14. Gender
15. Socioeconomic status
16. Symptoms
17. Type of physique

Hospital Variables

1. Drug therapy
2. Duration of hospitalization
3. Family therapy
4. Group therapy
5. Hours per week of psychotherapy
6. Improvement at discharge
7. Length of psychotherapy sessions
8. Level of function at discharge
9. Mode of treatment of schizophrenia: Insulin vs. psychotherapy
10. Number of family visits
11. Parental therapy
12. Participation in student government
13. Prognosis at discharge
14. Response to psychotherapy
15. School attendance
16. Use of day-hospital program

Posthospital Variables

1. Ability to relate to family
2. Following recommendations made at time of discharge
3. Length of interval between discharge and follow-up

2) The influence of these innovations fades quickly following discharge.
3) Aftercare clinics and other types of supportive aftercare services reduce recidivism significantly. It is unclear, however, whether the positive effects are due to medication, the provision of additional services, or the type of patients who use aftercare services.
4) Transitional facilities (i.e., halfway houses and partial hospitalization programs) also reduce recidivism, but fail to influence posthospital employment.

In a monumental survey of outcome studies of hospitalized adults, Erickson[11] concludes (in agreement with Anthony et al.[3]) that it is easier to shorten patients' hospital lengths of stay than it is to decrease posthospital recidivism or increase productive employment. Erickson agrees that almost any reasonable innovation can be shown to improve patient behavior in a hospital setting and shorten the length of stay. He emphasizes that these studies take place in the cultural context of a move away from large, long-term, custodial care institutions toward smaller, more active treatment institutions. Although this development is desirable, Erickson demonstrates conclusively that it can go too far. That is, if one defines hospital *efficiency* in terms of shorter lengths of stay, and defines hospital *effectiveness* as reduced recidivism and increased productive employment, current adult outcome research data demonstrate that drastically shortened lengths of stay lead directly to poor posthospital community function, reduced employment rates, and higher recidivism (the "revolving-door" syndrome). Erickson concludes,

> In the final analysis, however, there is only one finally defensible set of outcome measures—those which assess the patients' functioning in the community at follow-up.

In that regard, two general sets of factors emerge from the follow-up studies of adults reviewed both by Anthony et al.[3] and Erickson[11] that significantly improve patients' posthospital levels of satisfaction, employment, symptomatology, and interpersonal functioning. They are:

1) "Unitization" of hospital treatment facilities to include moving away from large, bureaucratic hospitals with centralized authority and low staff-patient ratios to hospital treatment services provided through relatively small living units with high staff-patient ratios, decentralized authority, decisions shared by various levels of staff, and maximal patient participation in planning programs and in decisions. Such semi-autonomous units eliminate routine ward transfers; therefore, "back wards" as well.

2) Provision of effective supportive aftercare services to include monitoring of medication, outpatient psychotherapy, educational and vocational guidance, training in social skills, and the use of appropriate transitional facilities such as halfway houses and partial hospitalization programs.

OVERVIEW OF LITERATURE

Combining the findings of the adolescent and adult studies, recommendations emerge for treatment program planning and for treatment evaluation research. In the area of *program planning,* the following steps are recommended.

1) The clinical decision-maker should support the development of innovative treatment approaches rather than relying solely on traditional ones. Because almost all "reasonable" treatment innovations seem to improve patients' *hospital* behavior, and this improvement is a valuable and legitimate goal, innovative approaches are definitely in order. Research data suggest that valuable approaches to innovation would be those that deal directly with the special needs of special groups. For example, programs attending to the particular developmental needs of children, adolescents, young adults, and older adults will likely augment treatment outcome. In addition, innovative programs oriented specifically toward clinical syndromes of greatest severity and chronicity are sorely needed, as well as special programs for patients with below average intellectual abilities. Teaching social and vocational skills directly to those with lower intellectual capabilities or chronic profound psychopathology is a promising area. Finally, innovative programs designed to elicit and maintain maximum family sup-

port for the identified patient after discharge are also encouraged by the research literature.

2) Hospital systems still utilizing ward transfers or large treatment units are well advised to follow the proven changes to smaller, semi-autonomous, decision-sharing treatment units.

3) Responsible hospital treatment does not stop at the time of discharge. The adequate provision of aftercare psychotherapy, social and vocational skill training, educational and vocational guidance, medications, and transitional living and treatment facilities clearly influence long-term outcome. A special focus on the development and maintenance of vocational capabilities is clearly in order.

Turning to issues of *evaluation study,* research efforts at this time might well focus on refinement of the known measures of variables that correlate with successful outcome to increase their predictive accuracy.[10] The data also support the development of more sophisticated and clinically relevant multivariate approaches in which the relationships of combinations of variables to treatment outcome are examined. This approach promises to increase understanding of the interactions between various patient, family, and treatment variables and how they influence long-term outcome. In this way, the state of the art can be moved closer to being able to provide the treatment modalities most helpful to patients with different types of syndromes, thus improving effectiveness of treatment.

REFERENCES

1. Aarkrog, T., Lauritsen, S., Mortensen, K., & Strom, J. Adolescents in psychiatric residential treatment and five years later. *Acta Psychiatric Scandinavica,* 1979, Supplement 278, Copenhagen.
2. Annesley, P., Psychiatric illness in adolescence: Presentation and prognosis. *Journal of Mental Science,* 1961, *107,* 268–278.
3. Anthony, W., Buell, G., Sharratt, S., & Althoff, M. Efficacy of psychiatric rehabilitation. *Psychological Bulletin,* 1972, *78,* 447–456.
4. Beavers, W., & Blumberg, S. A follow-up study of adolescents treated in an inpatient setting. *Diseases of the Nervous System,* 1968, *29,* 606–612.
5. Beckett, P., Pearson, C., & Rubin, E. A follow-up study comparing two approaches to the inpatient treatment of adolescent boys. *Journal of Nervous and Mental Disease,* 1962, *134,* 330–338.

6. Beskind, H. Psychiatric inpatient treatment of adolescents: A review of clinical experience. *Comprehensive Psychiatry,* 1962, *3,* 354–369.
7. Cameron, K., Bardon, D., & Mackeith, S. Symposium on the inpatient treatment of psychotic adolescents. *British Journal of Medical Psychology,* 1950, *23,* 107–118.
8. Carter, A. The prognostic factors of adolescent psychoses. *Journal of Mental Science,* 1942, *88,* 31–81.
9. Clarizio, H. Stability of deviant behavior through time. *Mental Hygiene,* 1968, *52,* 288–293.
10. Davis, D., Gonzalez, V., & Piat, J. Follow-up adolescent psychiatric patients. *Southern Medical Journal,* 1980, *73* (9), 1215–1218.
11. Erickson, R. Outcome studies in mental hospitals: A review. *Psychological Bulletin,* 1975, *82,* 519–540.
12. Garber, B. *Follow-up Study of Hospitalized Adolescents.* New York: Brunner/Mazel, 1972.
13. Garmezy, N. Process and reactive schizophrenia: Some conceptions and issues. *Schizophrenia Bulletin,* 1970, *2,* 30–74.
14. Gossett, J., Barnhart, D., Lewis, J., & Phillips, V. Follow-up of adolescents treated in a psychiatric hospital: Predictors of outcome. *Archives of General Psychiatry,* 1977, *34,* 1037–1042.
15. Gossett, J., Lewis, S., Lewis, J., & Phillips, V. Follow-up of adolescents treated in a psychiatric hospital: A review of studies. *American Journal of Orthopsychiatry,* 1973, *43,* 602–610.
16. Grob, M., & Singer, J. *Adolescent Patients in Transition: Impact and Outcome of Psychiatric Hospitalization.* New York: Behavioral Publications, 1974.
17. Groeschel, B. Social adjustment after residential treatment. In D. F. Ricks, A. Thomas, & M. Roff (Eds.), *Life History Research in Psychopathology,* (Vol. 3). Minneapolis: University of Minnesota Press, 1974, pp. 259–274.
18. Hafner, A., Quast, W., & Shea, J. The adult adjustment of 1000 psychiatric and pediatric patients: Initial findings from a 25-year follow-up. In R. D. Wirt, G. Winokur, & M. Roff, (Eds.), *Life History Research in Psychopathology,* (Vol. 4). Minneapolis: University of Minnesota Press, 1975, pp. 167–186.
19. Hartmann, E., Glasser, B., Greenblatt, M., Solomon, M., & Levinson, D. *Adolescents in a Mental Hospital.* New York: Grune & Stratton, 1968. (The same patient sample was described again in a subsequent paper: Herrera, E., Lifson, B., Hartmann, E., & Solomon, M. A 10-year follow-up of 55 hospitalized adolescents. *American Journal of Psychiatry,* 1974, *131,* 769–774).
20. Higgins, J. The concept of process-reactive schizophrenia: Criteria and related research. *Journal of Nervous and Mental Disease,* 1968, *138,* 9–25.
21. Higgins, J. Process-reactive schizophrenia: Recent developments. In R. Cancro (Ed.), *The Schizophrenic Syndrome: An Annual Review.* New York: Brunner/Mazel, 1971.
22. Kantor, R., & Herron, W. *Reactive and Process Schizophrenia.* Palo Alto: Science and Behavior Books, 1966.
23. King, L., & Pittman, G. A six-year follow-up study of sixty-five adolescent patients: Predictive value of presenting clinical picture. *British Journal of Psychiatry,* 1969, *115,* 1437–1441.
24. Kivowitz, J., Forgotson, J., Golstein, G., & Gottlieb, F. A follow-up study of hos-

pitalized adolescents. *Comprehensive Psychiatry,* 1974, *15* (1), 35–41.
25. Levy, E. Long-term follow-up of former inpatients at the Children's Hospital of the Menninger Clinic. *American Journal of Psychiatry,* 1969, *125,* 1633–1693.
26. Masterson, J. Prognosis in adolescent disorders. *American Journal of Psychiatry,* 1958, *114,* 1097–1103.
27. Masterson, J. Prognosis in adolescent disorders: Schizophrenia. *Journal of Nervous and Mental Disease,* 1956, *124,* 219–232.
28. Masterson, J., & Costello, J. L. *From Borderline Adolescent to Functioning Adult: The Test of Time.* New York: Brunner/Mazel, 1980.
29. Offer, D., Marcus, D., & Offer, J. A longitudinal study of normal adolescent boys. *American Journal of Psychiatry,* 1970, *126,* 917–924.
30. Pollack, M., Levenstein, S., & Klein, D. A three-year post-hospital follow-up of adolescent and adult schizophrenics. *American Journal of Orthopsychiatry,* 1968, *38,* 94–109.
31. Renaud, H., & Estess, F. Life history interviews with one hundred normal American males: "Pathogenicity" of childhood. *American Journal of Orthopsychiatry,* 1961, *31,* 786–802.
32. Roff, M. Childhood social interactions and young adult bad conduct. *Journal of Abnormal Social Psychology,* 1961, *63,* 333–337.
33. Schofield, W. & Balian, L. A comparative study of the personal histories of schizophrenic and non-psychiatric patients. *Journal of Abnormal Social Psychology,* 1959, *59,* 216–255.
34. Warren, W. A study of adolescent psychiatric in-patients and the outcome six or more years later: II—The follow-up study. *Journal of Child Psychology and Psychiatry,* 1965, *6,* 141–160.
35. Welner, A., Welner, Z., & Fishman, R. Psychiatric adolescent inpatients: Eight to ten-year follow-up. *Archives of General Psychiatry,* 1979, *36,* 687–700.
36. Zigler, E., & Phillips, F. Social competence and outcome in psychiatric disorder. *Journal of Abnormal & Social Psychology,* 1961, *63,* 264–271.
37. Zigler, E., & Phillips, F. Social competence and the Process-Reactive distinction in psychopathology. *Journal of Abnormal and Social Psychology,* 1962, *65,* 215–222.

CHAPTER 3

Development of the Research Project: The Pilot Studies

THE HOSPITAL SETTING

The hospital in which this study was conducted is a private psychiatric facility which has been in existence for 65 years. It is located on 27 acres in what is now a suburban residential area. The grounds are wooded and look like a college campus. The 168 hospital beds are distributed among seven semi-autonomous treatment units located in four single-story brick buildings. Additional buildings house administrative offices, a school, recreational and occupational therapy departments, a cafeteria, professionals' offices, and associated maintenance structures. A separate research and educational foundation is located on adjacent property.

The treatment philosophy is psychotherapeutic, and a variety of such therapies are used. The basic ideology is psychoanalytic, although a broader systems orientation is clearly demonstrated by the important role played by small-group theory and marital and family therapy. There is emphasis on interdisciplinary treatment teams, and all the traditional mental health professions are present. Leadership, however, is clearly psychiatric in that each treatment team is led by a psychiatrist, and the hospital governing board is comprised of senior psychiatrists only. A therapist-administrator split is used, with each patient having an administrative psychiatrist and an individual therapist. The therapist may be a psychiatrist, a clinical psychologist, or a psychiatric resident. The final responsibility for each patient's management is clearly vested in the administrative psychiatrist, although he or she consults frequently with the patient's therapist. The staff is closed, but psychiatrists or psychologists from the community may continue to function as therapists with patients whom they have referred to the hospital. The hospital also operates a day hospital, transitional living house, and an apartment living project.

There is strong educational emphasis. The hospital has an approved four-year residency program with 20 residents and is a site for the clerkship in psychiatry for students at the local medical school. In addition, the hospital has numerous university affiliations, including several schools of nursing which send students for a psychiatric rotation. Graduate students from two schools of social work, occupational therapy students, recreational therapy students, and others comprise the large body of students who receive all or part of their psychiatric training at the hospital.

One of the four inpatient clinical services is the Child and Adolescent Service. Currently this service is made up of three units: a boys' adolescent unit, a girls' adolescent unit, and a children's unit. The Adolescent Service began in the early 1960s and originally cared for adolescent patients who were housed with the adult population. In 1968 the adolescent patients moved to separate units, and the children's unit was added in 1980.

THE ADOLESCENT PATIENTS

Most of the patients on the Adolescent Service are from middle- and upper-middle class families, and their hospital fees are supported significantly by hospital insurance. The reputation of the Adolescent Service for providing intermediate- and long-term intensive, reconstructive treatment encourages referrals from local, regional, and national sources, and there is often a waiting list. These factors influence the nature and severity of the psychopathology of the patients admitted, who, by and large, are seriously disturbed teenagers, and most often the disturbances are chronic. With rare exceptions, the patients have had earlier treatment; prior outpatient psychotherapy and one or more prior hospitalizations are the rule.

The patients represent the full spectrum of severe diagnostic categories, but most commonly, severe character or personality disorders. Currently, many of these patients would be diagnosed borderline personality.

The second most common diagnosis is schizophrenia, and most patients are admitted after the stage of acute psychosis. They are seen as either chronic or moving toward chronicity.

There is also a smaller group of patients admitted to the Adolescent Service with severe and incapacitating phobic or dysthymic disturbances coupled with milder personality disorders; before DSM-III, such patients were referred to as experiencing a severe neurotic disorder.

THE TREATMENT PROGRAM

Although there are differences in the content, style, and temporal patterning of each adolescent's treatment program, there are major features likely to exist at any given time for most patients. For descriptive purposes, these may be divided into three general areas: the treatment milieu, the school, and the psychotherapies.

Treatment Milieu

At the core of an effective treatment program an ambience will be noted that is relatively easy to perceive but difficult to describe. The adequacy of the physical plant, the architecture and decor of the buildings, and the attractiveness of the grounds play a part, but more than all else the ambience represents the quality of feeling tone created by staff and patients in thousands of daily interpersonal transactions. The administrative psychiatrist in charge of the unit makes a substantial contribution to the ambience through his or her style of directing, confronting, and nurturing. However, the nursing personnel may have the greatest impact on the milieu through their role in the day-to-day operations of the unit. When nursing personnel relate to each other and to the patients with clear communications and flexibility, negotiating decisions when appropriate, showing confident optimism, respect, empathy, and demonstrating the capacity to be authoritative if demanded by the circumstances, there is great likelihood that what has been called a "protreatment group process" will evolve on the unit.[6] Under these circumstances, patients and staff can work together toward shared therapeutic goals.

The prevailing psychoanalytic perspective regarding each patient's dilemma is augmented by a major concern with the quality of the group process on each unit. Because patients have profound impact on each other, either for better or worse, creating a milieu in which there is maximum opportunity for positive patient-to-patient influence is seen as crucial to the success of patients' treatment plans.

The involvement of several staff members in family systems research growing out of this treatment evaluation project has provided additional theoretical constructs with which to understand the unit social system.[5] In particular, the ability to distinguish social system characteristics that influence individual growth and autonomy has been helpful.[7]

The Hospital School

A common characteristic of successful adolescent treatment programs is the existence of a hospital school to meet the patients' educational needs (see Chapter 2). While the course content may resemble that of schools from which the patients come and to which some will return, the style of the educational experience differs dramatically. There is a staff commitment to the idea that the work of adolescence is education. As a consequence, even severely disturbed youngsters are in the classroom, and classes are small (6-10 students). Because the demands on the teachers to tolerate disturbed behavior, to relate with both empathy and firmness, and to maintain reasonable educational objectives are heavy, the school's most important asset is a cadre of unusually skilled and dedicated teachers.

The Psychotherapies

All patients who remain hospitalized beyond the initial weeks of evaluation have individual psychotherapy twice weekly or, in some instances, more frequently. Most patients are seen by experienced therapists, although a small number are assigned to a second-, third-, or fourth-year resident. Considerable effort is made to "match" patient and therapist. Much of the matching is intuitive, although a number of the experienced therapists have particular skills with specific types of psychopathology. The psychotherapy is clearly psychoanalytic in orientation.

All but the most profoundly disturbed patients are engaged also in a twice-a-week coed group psychotherapeutic experience. This treatment modality is provided in addition to the daily unit meetings in which there also occurs a variety of therapeutic processes such as confrontation, emotional support, and clarification.

Most patients also participate in family therapy. Although the parents are often involved actively in the treatment process from the time of admission, formal family therapy usually does not begin until that point in the treatment process at which the patient has worked through initial resistances to treatment.

Patients work through significant psychological conflicts in individual psychotherapy, group psychotherapy, daily unit meetings, and family therapy which focus on material provided by the patients' interactions on the units and in school. In turn, insights derived from these treatment processes are shared with the unit staff and school personnel in terms useful to those settings. Because many patients may have three therapists (individual, group, and family), many hours of interdisciplinary staff meetings each week are needed to share clinical data, formulate or reformulate clinical hypotheses, and plan interventions.

BACKGROUND

In July, 1966, the Adolescent Service underwent major reorganization and expansion. As one part of this change, a commitment to treatment evaluation and follow-up was established. The reasons for this were multiple and included the staff's interest in improving the quality of their work; the adverse impact on staff morale of hearing informal reports about "bad" outcomes (marginal community adjustments, rehospitalization, and suicide); and scientific curiosity. During the initial 18 months, the treatment team met periodically to plan formal follow-up procedures.

The First and Second Pilot Projects

In 1968, the staff had a day-long conference in which outcome data regarding the 35 patients who had been discharged since July 1966 were shared. These patients had been out of the hospital for periods ranging from one to 18 months. Although every former patient was interviewed, no systematic measures were used, and outcome levels of function were assessed informally. After 18 months, an additional 21 patients had been discharged, and a second conference was held.

Over the years of these early efforts, the project assumed a different form. Initially, the major focus was on how well or poorly the discharged patients were doing. Extreme variability in levels of functioning from patient to patient during the first year after discharge was noted in both 1968 and 1969. This observation led naturally to the need to follow these patients for a longer period and increased interest in those factors that might explain differences in treatment outcome. As the literature about hospital treatment follow-up was explored, it became apparent that certain key variables needed to be examined in greater detail. Although earlier studies demonstrate that several variables are powerful correlates of treatment outcome, no quantified scales existed with which to measure these variables. Work began on developing refined measures of severity of patient psychopathology (see Chapter 6 and Appendix A), and family level of competence (see Chapter 6 and Appendix C).

The Third Pilot Project

The third pilot project data (1970–1972) will be presented in summary form in this chapter. The 56 patients studied previously had been discharged for periods ranging from 20–48 months. During their hospitalization, there were usually 25 adolescent patients in the hospital, and they were distributed throughout six living units along with adult patients.

Of the 56 patients, 14 were profoundly disturbed and received psychotropic medications during most or all of their hospitalization (range of 78–359 medication days, median 157 days). Another group of 11 patients received medication only during periods of severe disturbance (range of 1–50 medication days, median 14 days). The remainder received no major psychotropic medications. The policy of using medication only when interpersonal support was insufficient resulted in only the more profoundly disturbed patients receiving medications. As a consequence, the impact of medication upon treatment outcome was not independent of severity of psychopathology.

Follow-up data were obtained on 55 of the 56 patients. At the time of admission they were between 13 and 19 years (with an average of 16 years); 24 were boys and 31 were girls. Of the 55 patients, 11 were discharged after evaluation, and the remaining 44 were hospitalized from 1–17 months (median 7 months). As a group, they were primarily white, middle-class, and Protestant. Diagnoses were: 31 personality disorder; 14 psychosis; and 10 severe neurosis. Nearly all were admitted following the failure of prior outpatient and inpatient treatment efforts.

Several measures to be used in a systematic way were developed.

Severity of Psychopathology

The severity of patient psychopathology was evaluated by consensus of the treatment team in terms of neurotic, personality disorder, or psychotic functioning. While this three-level categorization represents gross evaluations, prior studies demonstrate that the average level of psychopathology between these diagnostic categories differs (see Chapter 2).

Onset of Symptomatology

The label "process" refers to those forms of psychopathology that appear to have symptomatic origin in the earliest years of life, evolving slowly over a number of years into deeply internalized life patterns. Those labeled "reactive" appear to be more recent symptomatic responses associated with ongoing stress. The Onset of Symptomatology Scale (Appendix B) quantifies clinical judgments on this continuum by measurement on seven subscales. Literature review suggests that the most promising dimensions are academic failure, peer isolation, marked passivity, slow treatment response, and early, gradual, and bland development of symptoms. Review of our patients' charts, however, revealed inadequate data were available for assessing rate of symptom onset, intensity of onset, and early treatment response. Therefore, subscales for academic progress, peer relationships, passivity, and duration of symptoms were developed. In addition, though less well supported by prior research, subscales were derived for early psychological trauma, early physical trauma, and "oddness" or behavioral peculiarities in early childhood.[3]

Scores on the seven subscales were summed, with the total score being used to place each patient (regardless of diagnosis) on the process-reactive continuum. A psychiatrist* experienced in treating children and adolescents—and unfamiliar with the patient sample—read the initial hospital chart and rated each patient on the seven-part Onset of Symptomatology Scale. Interrater reliability between this judge and one of the investigators (JTG) was .79 (linear correlation coefficient, $p < .001$). Patients scoring on the lower half of the scale range were categorized *reactive,* with those in the upper half being called *process.*

Assaultiveness

Several staff members had observed that patients whose behavior prior to hospitalization had not involved appreciable physical threat to others seemed to have a better treatment course than those who had been physically destructive or threatening to others. After reviewing historical information on each patient (but prior to the review of follow-up information), the clinical team made a consensual judgment of the degree of physically destructive and threatening behavior engaged in prior to hospitalization on a five-point scale: None, Mild, Moderate, Severe, and Profound.

---

*John E. Meeks, M.D.

Energy Level

Other clinical impressions suggested that treatment of those patients generally described as extremely lethargic, apathetic, or profoundly passive was much less successful than those of average or above-average energy and activity levels. In arriving at a staff consensus concerning the patient's typical level of physical energy, every attempt was made to disregard the productivity or lack of productivity of the activity, the relative appropriateness of the activity level, or speculations concerning the psychodynamics underlying activity level. This conceptualization was derived in part from the contributions of Thomas, Chess, and Birch[12] and, in part, from clinical observations that the treatment team was more successful in encouraging energetic youngsters to channel their vitality into more productive pursuits than they were in assisting lethargic patients to be more energetic. Energy level was rated as Above Average, Average, or Below Average (compared to "normal"). These ratings also were made following a staff review of patient history, but before knowledge of follow-up data.

Type of Treatment Termination

For this analysis, inpatient treatment termination consisted of two categories derived by consensus of the treatment team at time of discharge: inpatient treatment incomplete or complete.

Continuation of Psychotherapy

Continuation of individual psychotherapy after discharge was recommended for all patients. Responses to this recommendation were classified as: psychotherapy discontinued at the time of hospital discharge; psychotherapy continued intermittently after discharge, without mutually agreed upon termination; or psychotherapy continued after discharge to mutually agreed upon completion.

Responsibility for the follow-up of each patient was given to one of the three psychiatrists or two psychologists who had the most meaningful relationship with the ex-patient.* Approximately equal num-

---

*Doyle I. Carson, M.D., John T. Gossett, Ph.D., Joe W. King, M.D., Jerry M. Lewis, M.D., and Dale R. Turner, Ph.D.

bers of patients were assigned to each of the five follow-up investigators.

The goals and procedures of the follow-up investigation were discussed with patients and parents on several occasions during hospitalization. This information was reviewed with each patient and the parents prior to follow-up interview, at which time his or her consent was obtained.

Although the style of interviewing varied, each investigator obtained a face-to-face contact whenever possible; otherwise telephone calls were relied on. The investigators obtained information in the following areas: 1) current living situation; 2) peer relationships; 3) current symptoms; 4) current drug and alcohol usage; 5) legal difficulties; 6) academic functioning; 7) work adjustment; 8) subjective contentment; 9) parents' and/or spouse's evaluation (obtained directly); 10) plans for the next few years; and 11) outpatient and/or inpatient treatment following discharge.

This follow-up information was presented by the interviewer at a staff meeting. The staff discussed the patient's progress and made a consensual judgment of the patient's degree of improvement and level of function. Improvement was evaluated as Marked, Moderate, Some, None, or Worse, as compared to status at admission. Level of function in the community (as compared impressionistically to other youngsters of the same age, sex, intelligence, and socioeconomic status) was evaluated as Good, Fair, or Poor. Those youngsters living productive lives without evidence of psychiatric impairment were rated Good. Those living productively but with some remaining problems were rated Fair. For the purposes of this report these two groups are combined as Adaptive. Poor ratings were given to those able to function only with continuing massive support from family or therapists, those currently or intermittently rehospitalized, and those unable to function in school, work, and interpersonal relationships.

An argument can be made for using either Improvement, Level of Function, or both to evaluate treatment outcome. Considering the severity of psychopathology of these patients and the fact that previous outpatient or inpatient treatment had been unsuccessful, any significant degree of improvement may be seen as worthwhile. Nevertheless, if improvement, however marked, leaves the expatient unable to function adequately, its accomplishment is, at best, a hollow success. The ratings of Improvement and Level of Function correlated .95. It seemed parsimonious, therefore, to select one rating as the standard of outcome. Level of Function was selected as being the more meaningful measure of the overall impact of treatment. It is both more conservative and relates most directly to the former patient's ability to function in the "real world." All patients arrived at the hospital at the same level (Poor), and changes on this measure offer an estimate of the realistic usefulness of inpatient treatment to the patient, the family, and to society.

Predictors of Outcome

Examination of the relationship of each predictor to Level of Function at outcome produces the results shown in Table 3.

All variables are related in the expected direction; for example, the 10 patients receiving neurotic diagnoses attained Adaptive outcome, while nine of the 14 psychotic patients functioned at a Poor level at follow-up. More than half of the patients with a personality disorder diagnosis had Adaptive outcome. Most of the patients achieving an Onset of Symptomatology score reflecting more recent symptomatic development were seen to be functioning adaptively at outcome, while 18 of the 33 with more chronic disorders were assessed at a Poor level at follow-up.

A majority of patients demonstrating no assaultiveness achieved Adaptive outcome (19 of 25), while those with varying degrees of such behavior were distributed equally in outcome categories.

Most patients with average or above-average energy (73 percent) were functioning at an Adaptive level at follow-up, while those with below-average available energy divided evenly between Poor and Adaptive outcome. The majority of patients who completed the goals of the hospital treatment program and continued in recommended psychotherapy following discharge did well, while those who did not complete the hospital treatment plan and discontinued psychotherapy at the time of discharge or shortly thereafter again divided evenly between outcome categories.

TABLE 3

Relationship Between Predictors and Level of Function at Follow-Up

Variable	n	Level of Function	
		Adaptive	Poor
Diagnosis			
Neurosis	10	10	0
Personality Disorder	31	19	12
Psychosis	14	5	9
$X^2 = 10.3, p < .005$			
Onset of Symptomatology			
Reactive (0–13)	22	19	3
Process (14–24)	33	15	18
$X^2 = 7.7, p < .005$			
Assaultiveness			
None	25	19	6
Mild to Profound	30	15	15
$X^2 = 2.88, p < .05$			
Energy Level			
Above Average	18	12	6
Average	15	12	3
Below Average	22	10	12
$X^2 = 4.7, p < .05$			
Hospital Treatment			
Completed	14	12	2
Incomplete	41	22	19
$X^2 = 5.59, p < .01$			
Psychotherapy Following Discharge			
Continued	12	10	2
Intermittent	28	18	10
None	15	6	9
$X^2 = 5.5, p < .05$			

Combining Outcome Predictors

To evaluate the usefulness of retaining or dropping each of the predictor variables when using them in combination, regression analysis was performed using the significant variables (Table 4).[4]

This analysis suggests that diagnostic severity has the most predictive power and that meaningful additions can be obtained by using four of the other five variables (assaultiveness did not add to the multiple regression analysis).

The complex interrelationships among the predictor variables and the outcome measure can be illustrated in diagrammatic form as shown in Figure 1. To simplify the diagram, average and above-average Energy Level have been combined and labeled High to contrast with below average energy; Intermittent and Completed Posthospital Psychotherapy have been combined as Continued; and Good and Fair outcome have been combined and labeled Adaptive.

Figure 1 can be entered at any level for an analysis of the impact of a given variable on outcome and an understanding of the relationship of that variable to the other predictors. For example, when entering the diagram at the level of Diagnostic Severity, it is seen that the 10 neurotic patients were functioning well at follow-up, regardless of their Process-Reactive Onset scores, Energy Level, Type of Treatment Termination, or Continuation of Psychotherapy after discharge. Most psychotic patients (nine of 14) were functioning poorly at follow-up regardless of

TABLE 4

Step-wise Multiple Regression Summary

| | | Multiple | | |
| | | | | Increase |
Step No.	Variable	R	R²	in R²
1.	Diagnostic severity	.44	.19	.19
2.	Treatment termination	.51	.26	.07
3.	Energy level	.55	.30	.04
4.	Posthospital therapy	.59	.34	.04
5.	Onset of symptomatology	.62	.38	.04

Note. Dependent variable equals follow-up level of function. Follow-up level of function equals .56 + .33 diagnostic severity plus .22 energy level plus .33 onset of symptomatology plus .29 termination plus .25 posthospital therapy.

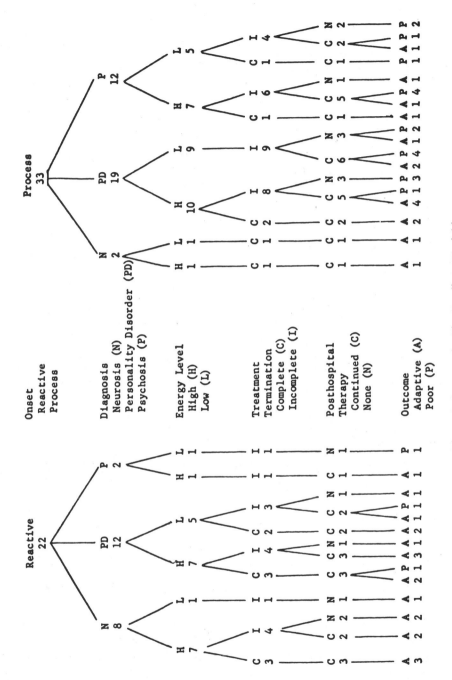

Figure 1. Outcome by Five Predictor Variables

45

their location on other measures. However, for the five psychotic patients who were functioning well at follow-up, four were average or above average in Energy Level and four continued in psychotherapy after discharge.

Among the personality disorder patients, those seen as Reactive tended to function better at follow-up (10 of 12 were Adaptive outcome), as compared to those of a Process type (nine of 19 with Adaptive outcome). Among the Process personality disorder patients, most with Adaptive outcome (six of nine) were of average or above-average Energy Level and two of the remaining three low Energy Level, Process personality disorder patients who did well continued in psychotherapy after hospital discharge.

COMMENT

Patient and treatment variables related to long-term outcome do not function in isolation from one another. Previous adolescent treatment outcome studies suffer from the failure to develop data indicating anything about the interactions among such variables. The single earlier study including a serious attempt at multivariate analysis is the follow-up reported by Garber.[2] The overall results of this unusually well designed and executed study support earlier findings of the importance of patients' initial severity of psychopathology and focus on the long-term significance of patients' relationship skills. Unfortunately, the multivariate portion of their analysis does not yield additional information. This may well be due to their use of the Automatic Interaction Detection Technique (AID), a statistical approach designed for large-sample, survey data. Their sample consists of only 120 cases (which they further divided into two random subsets of 60 cases each). Instructions for the use of AID suggest the technique should be restricted to data sets of a thousand or more cases.[11]

Meehl and Rosen[8] argue persuasively that the usual methods of prediction in clinical research are inadequate unless one considers the natural rates of occurrence of the phenomena being predicted, the type of clinical populations being examined, and the restrictive impact of small sample sizes. With these cautions, the results of this Pilot Study are to be considered tentative and suggestive rather than definitive. We do not know, for example, the levels of function that would naturally occur for such youngsters if no treatment were provided. Long-term follow-up studies of adolescents with personality disorder and psychotic level psychopathology receiving little or no treatment are rare, but suggest more "spontaneous deterioration"[1] than "spontaneous remission."[9,10]

Despite these difficulties, several tentative generalizations may be offered. The strongest admission predictors of long-term outcome continue to be those associated with severity of the patient's psychopathology and those that differentiate recent from long-term psychiatric dysfunction. These factors, however, are not independent but appear to have a consistent pattern of interaction.

Patients diagnosed as neurotic have a high probability of being evaluated as functioning well several years after hospital discharge, regardless of the duration of the symptoms prior to hospitalization. Patients given a diagnosis of process or chronic psychosis during adolescence have a low probability of being able to function well several years after hospital treatment, although a small number do recover. High energy level and continuation of psychotherapy after hospital discharge seem to contribute to these uncommon recoveries.

Patients who experience psychotic or personality disorder symptoms of shorter duration (reactive) generally have adaptive long-term outcomes, although a small number begin to appear chronic in young adulthood.

Patients with many years of personality disorder symptomatology have very mixed outcomes, and attempts to define more specific predictors for this group have not yet succeeded. Within this group of long-term, or process, personality disorders, future investigators may profitably examine patient, family, and treatment variables in greater depth. Among the 19 such patients in the Pilot Study, nine had an Adaptive outcome, while 10 were functioning at a Poor level at follow-up. Neither energy level nor the type of treatment termination helped predict outcome within this group. A tentative lead for future exploration, however, may be noted in the finding that, of the six patients within the process personality disorder group who terminated psychotherapy at the time of hospital discharge, five had Poor long-term outcome, while eight of 13 who continued with their therapists after hospital discharge were functioning at an Adaptive level at follow-up. The examination of additional variables and combinations of variables did not yield further helpful clues.

The results of this Pilot project concur with earlier follow-up studies: Severity of psychopathology and the type of onset of symptomatology are powerful predictors of long-term outcome. Several other variables also correlated with outcome. To some degree, these correlations are independent of severity and onset; that is, patients across a wide range of severity and chronicity of disorder with high average available energy, who complete recommended inpatient treatment and who continue in psychotherapy following hospital discharge, tend to have better long-term function than those who possess low levels of energy, leave the hospital prematurely, or terminate psychotherapy at the time of discharge.

During the early years of this research project, the study was conducted by the staff of the Adolescent Service without outside funding. By 1968 two of the clinicians had assumed research positions part-time, and in 1970 funding was obtained for a five-year period. The clinically useful results of this Pilot Project, and the availability of funding, provided the opportunity for two key clinicians to become part-time clinical investigators and led to a more detailed, full-scale follow-up project.

REFERENCES

1. Bergin, A. E., & Suinn, R. M. Individual psychotherapy and behavior therapy. *Annual Review of Psychology,* 1975, *26,* 509–556.
2. Garber, B. *Follow-up Study of Hospitalized Adolescents.* New York: Brunner/Mazel, 1972.
3. Gossett, J. T., Meeks, J. E., Barnhart, F. D., & Phillips, V. A. Follow-up of adolescents treated in a psychiatric hospital: The onset of symptomatology scale. *Adolescence,* 1976, *11,* 195–211.
4. Labovitz, S. The assignment of numbers to rank order categories. *American Sociological Review,* 1970, *35* (3), 515–524.
5. Lewis, J. M., Beavers, W. R., Gossett, J. T., & Phillips, V. A. *No Single Thread: Psychological Health in Family Systems.* New York: Brunner/Mazel, 1976.
6. Lewis, J. M., Gossett, J. T., King, J. W., & Carson, D. I. Development of a protreatment group process among hospitalized adolescents. In S. Feinstein & P. Giovacchini (Eds.), *Adolescent Psychiatry: Developmental and Clinical Studies,* (Vol. 2). New York: Basic Books, 1973, pp. 351–362.
7. Looney, J. G., Blotcky, J. M., Carson, D. I., & Gossett, J. T. A family systems

model for inpatient treatment of adolescents. In S. Feinstein, P. Giovacchini, J. Looney, A. Schwartzberg, & A. Sorosky (Eds.), *Adolescent Psychiatry: Developmental and Clinical Studies,* (Vol. 8). Chicago: University of Chicago Press, 1980, pp. 499–511.

8. Meehl, P. E., & Rosen, A. Antecedent probability and the efficiency of psychometric signs, patterns, or cutting scores. *Psychological Bulletin,* 1955, *52* (3), 194–216.

9. Robins, L. N. *Deviant Children Grown Up.* Baltimore: Williams & Wilkins Co., 1966.

10. Shore, M. F., & Massimo, J. L. After ten years: A follow-up study of comprehensive vocationally oriented psychotherapy. *American Journal of Orthopsychiatry,* 1973, *43* (1), 128–132.

11. Sonquist, J. A., Baker, E. L., & Morgan, J. N. *Searching for Structure: An Approach to Analysis of Substantial Bodies of Micro-data and Documentation for a Computer Program.* Ann Arbor: University of Michigan, Institute for Social Research, 1971.

12. Thomas, A., Chess, S., & Birch, H. G. *Temperament and Behavior Disorders in Children.* New York: New York University Press, 1968.

PART II

The Main Study

CHAPTER 4

Measurement of Outcome

During the pilot stages of the Adolescent Treatment Assessment Project, much work was accomplished in developing scales for relevant patient, family, treatment process, and outcome variables. In this chapter we focus upon an overall outline of the full-scale follow-up study, emphasizing long-term patient outcome. In subsequent chapters we will integrate material relating to predictor variables.

METHODOLOGY

Sample

The outcome assessments presented here are based upon 120 consecutive admissions to the Timberlawn Hospital Adolescent Service between September 1968 and November 1972. The sample consists of 52 adolescent girls and 68 boys between the ages of 12 and 19 at the time of admission. Although 29 patients (24 percent) remained in the hospital less than six months, the majority remained from six to 24 months (median 13 months), and a small number, 14 (12 percent), were hospitalized for 25–45 months. The patients represent a variety of severe psychopathology, the majority suffering from impulse-ridden personality disorders. The symptoms most common prior to admission include se-

vere academic underachievement, drug and alcohol abuse, promiscuity, runaways, delinquent acts, severe and chronic conflict with authorities, and a failure to respond to prior treatment efforts. Although the
"borderline" diagnostic category was not in common use at the time
this patient sample was admitted, in retrospect it is clear that within
current diagnostic guidelines a large number of this sample could be re-
diagnosed as borderline syndromes. A subsample (approximately one-
quarter) presented with rather classical psychotic symptomatology,
primarily schizophrenic syndromes.

The last of the subject group was discharged from the hospital in
June 1974. Follow-up contacts began one year later.

Treatment Milieu

During the time of the Main Study, the adolescent girls resided in a
14-bed girls' unit, and the boys were housed nearby in a separate
12-bed unit. All patients lived in semi-private rooms and participated
in an intensive treatment milieu. This included a reality-based school
program; daily problem-solving meetings on the living units conducted
by the unit psychiatrists; individual, group, and family psychotherapy;
and a variety of athletic and activity programs, both on and off hospital grounds. The treatment philosophy clearly centered around the
concept of "treating people with people," although psychopharmaco-
logic agents were used where indicated. Unique characteristics of the
group process have been reported elsewhere.[4]

Follow-up Procedures

Prior work demonstrated that adjustment during the first year after
discharge tends to be quite variable for most patients. Thus, assessment during the initial post-discharge year is often unreliable (see Chapter 2). Since follow-up assessment for this patient group began in June
1975 and continued through September 1978, the time elapsed between the patients' hospital discharges and follow-up contacts ranges
from two years 11 months to seven years 8 months, with a median of
about five years.

Initial contact letters were mailed to former patients, requesting that they call us for a follow-up interview. If the former patient did not respond to the letter, a telephone contact was attempted. The senior author (JTG), who was well-known to the former patients, interviewed each of them, while another member of the assessment team (FDB) interviewed the former patients' parents. The interviews averaged 90 minutes in duration.

About half of the interviews were conducted face-to-face and the others by telephone. Although the majority of the personal interviews occurred at the Timberlawn Psychiatric Research Foundation, some were conducted (at their request) at the subjects' homes or apartments. Although face-to-face interviews were sought, this was often impossible because of geographic distance or, in some instances, the subject's preference. It is our opinion that telephone contacts, while providing less information, are nevertheless adequate for excellent follow-up assessment, especially when the interviewer is well-known to the former patient.

The format of the follow-up interview involves a reminder of the purposes of the study, obtaining informed consent, and an initial open-ended question requesting the subject to review the period between hospital discharge and the present. Following this, increasingly focused questions were asked relating to the former patient's friends, social life, romantic relationships, relationship with parents, educational and vocational history, physical health, patterns of usage of alcohol, marijuana, prescribed and nonprescribed drugs, contacts with legal authorities, and additional psychiatric treatment (see Appendix D).

A second portion of the interview focuses upon the subject's feelings about his or her hospital experience, including a description of those aspects felt to be most and least helpful. The interviewer notes any significant factors or special problems encountered during the interview and makes detailed notes concerning the subject's current appearance, style, and mental status.

This material is summarized in a written report, and the results of the interviews with the former patient and the parents are de-identified and combined in a Follow-up Folder.

Outcome Assessment

Two sets of judgments have been obtained, designed both to reflect the multidimensional nature of outcome and to provide ratings independent from the possible bias of treatment personnel. Three experienced mental health professionals from outside Timberlawn Psychiatric Center assessed follow-up Level of Function.* They read each patient's Follow-up Folder and made judgments for each on scales measuring: (a) peer and social function; (b) relationship with parents; and (c) educational and occupational functioning. The rating scales are presented in Table 5.

On each of these scales, a rating of "Good" suggests an essentially normal or healthy level of functioning with no evidence of impairment. "Fair" suggests that the former patient was functioning with some restriction or impairment related to psychiatric disability. "Poor" suggests inability to form meaningful and rewarding interpersonal or family relationships and the inability to function adequately educationally and occupationally on a regular basis. Ratings on the three basic scales —peer, family, and vocational function—were combined numerically to form an overall Global Level of Function. That is, the modal peer, family, and vocational score for each rater on each former patient was derived, and the modal figure based on the three raters for each subject was taken as a final Global Level of Function Score of 1 (Good), 2 (Fair), or 3 (Poor). Median scores were used when modes were not appropriate. Global ratings of Good and Fair are combined and labeled "Adaptive" for data analysis purposes.

Perhaps several vignettes will better explain the nature of Global Level of Function. These vignettes represent actual case histories, but names and other identifying facts have been changed to protect confidentiality.

Bill, 17 years old, was brought to the hospital by his parents in spite of very strong verbal and physical resistance. Bill denied any awareness of why he had been "dragged" to Timberlawn, but his parents de-

---

*Martin R. Gluck, Ph.D., Jack Martin, M.D., and Jean L. Roberts, M.D.

TABLE 5

Level of Function Scales

I. Peer and Social Functioning
1. *Good:* At least one intense, mutually gratifying relationship with a peer of either sex. Relationships with other peers of both sexes are not grossly restricted.
2. *Fair:* Clear evidence of marked restriction in some aspect of relationships with peers. Such restriction may be either that relations are superficial or that, despite having one intense relationship, there is some marked restriction as, for example, definitely impaired relationships with persons of the opposite sex.
3. *Poor:* No friends at all or only superficial acquaintances.

II. Relationship with Parents
1. *Good:* A stable relationship showing age-appropriate independence and demonstrating mutual respect and affection.
2. *Fair:* Relationship clearly impaired. (No attempt is made to assess how much of this might be attributable to the patient or the parents).
3. *Poor:* Relationship lacks all or most of the qualities rated *Good.*

III. Occupational Functioning
1. *Good:* Full-time, stable, and successful homemaking, employment, or school activity.
2. *Fair:* Only part-time involvement with homemaking, work, or school; or significant occupational problems such as truancy, acting out, underachievement, instability over time.
3. *Poor:* Unable or unwilling to perform occupational tasks on a regular basis.

scribed a history of behavioral difficulties dating back to early childhood. Bill's problems included belligerence at home, school failures beginning in the fourth grade, frequent vandalism, drug and alcohol abuse beginning in junior high school, and several arrests. Bill had his first psychological evaluation at age six, had been referred for outpatient psychotherapy at that time, and again while in junior high, and had been hospitalized for five weeks at a short-term psychiatric unit the year prior to the current admission. The current hospitalization was precipitated by a violent battle with his parents.

A highly intelligent and sometimes charming youngster, Bill vacillated from icy, controlling distance during much of his hospital stay, to brief periods of time in which he seemed more deeply involved with his peers, his individual psychotherapist, and other staff. After six months of hospitalization, however, at a time when the staff felt that Bill was beginning to make some genuine strides toward increasing maturity, he ran away from the hospital and persuaded his parents to allow him to return home.

Contacted by telephone in Indiana four years after discharge, Bill indicated that while he was not working at the time, he had held many jobs over the past several years. These primarily consisted of manual labor or transient sales work.

Bill had been married for approximately one-and-a-half years, but was separated at the time of our interview. Currently he was living with another young woman, but stated in a lackadaisical way that he was not very involved and certainly had no intention of marrying her. She was supporting him financially. Although still involved in drug use and occasional sales, Bill denied that he was "addicted" to any drug.

Bill indicated that he gets along well with his parents because he makes few demands on them. He continues from time to time to ask his father to help him when he has legal problems (which his father had done in the past, but currently refuses to do). Bill said, "They still bitch at me to get a job, but other than that, they stay off my back."

Bill's parents generally confirmed this report, emphasizing his vocational instability, continued difficulties with legal authorities, and inability to relate to peers except through shared antisocial activities or through using a succession of young women for economic support. Bill's parents agreed that they have virtually no contact with him since they began to refuse his requests for rescue from legal problems.

Bill was rated Poor on all outcome scales.

Barry, a tall, thin 16-year-old, was hospitalized in the midst of an acute psychotic reaction, secondary to hallucinogenic drug use. Three previous short-term hospitalizations following similar episodes had not led to more mature functioning. The only son of a lawyer and a schoolteacher, Barry had always been unusually shy and withdrawn. After beginning drug experimentation during the past year, his previous almost straight-A academic record had declined dramatically. Described as an "easy" young child by both of his parents, Barry's pronounced shyness and lack of friends had been the only area of parental concern prior to the past year.

When his more florid psychotic symptoms cleared, Barry expressed strong but mixed feelings about continued drug use. He readily acknowledged his inability to tolerate drugs (as evidenced by his psychotic episodes), but at the same time, he spoke movingly of drugs as a passport to friendships. Still very shy, awkward, and lonely, Barry confronted this conflict repeatedly during his eight months of hospitalization.

At the time of follow-up, Barry was a neatly groomed, quietly friendly 23-year-old. He described a period of intense loneliness following hospital discharge, which he gradually overcame through outpatient psychotherapy and involvement in college and church activities. Barry had regained his former high academic standing and was attending graduate school in a professional field. He had been able to establish several moderately close peer relationships and, at the present time, had a roommate whom he described as "a friend—not a real close friend, but at least a friend." Still hampered by extreme shyness, Barry had not been able to form a close relationship with a girl but remained hopeful that one day such a relationship would develop. Although Barry's past conflicts with his parents had abated, he described his current relationship with them as "respectful but distant."

Barry was given a rating of Good in the area of vocational functioning, Fair on the peer and parental scales, and a Global Level of Function of Adaptive.

Betty's entrance to the hospital was most dramatic. An attractive and highly energetic 14-year-old, she arrived in seductively revealing clothing and dominated the admission procedures with her aggressive style. Appearing on the surface to be in very good spirits, Betty's frequent loud laughter and numerous jokes thinly veiled her underlying anxiety. She behaved in a flirtatious manner with the young male admitting psychiatrist and seemed to enjoy regaling him with lurid exploits from her past. Her parents, by marked contrast, appeared exhausted and irritable, arguing frequently over details of their daughter's history.

Although it was difficult to obtain an organized account from Betty (or from the parents), it gradually became clear that she had a long history of running away from home (making it all the way to California on one occasion) and numerous wrist-cutting episodes, which she described as suicide attempts, but her parents labeled disparagingly as "manipulations." She had no girlfriends, but "many, many boyfriends." Although only 14, Betty had already experienced numerous sexual affairs and proudly claimed to have had intercourse "over 100 times." A very bright girl, she had failed repeatedly in school. Betty was transferred from an acute psychiatric unit of a general hospital where it was determined that she and her parents were in need of long-term work.

The early months of Betty's hospitalization were stormy, marked by extreme verbal resistance to treatment and two runaways. She was seductive with male staff and contemptuous of female staff. Unpopular with her better functioning hospital peers, she nevertheless became the leader of a group of highly resistant patients.

By the seventh month of hospital treatment, however, her defenses crumbled, and the frightened, depressed, childlike core of her personality emerged. As Betty shared her deeper feelings and conflicts more openly with her therapist, peers, unit staff, and with her parents in family therapy, issues that had long remained hidden began to emerge and be resolved.

Betty began attending a public school off hospital grounds and visiting with her parents every weekend. In spite of several relapses into acting-out behavior, her overall level of maturity continued to improve and, after 14 months of hospitalization, she returned home.

At the time of follow-up, Betty was a slender, very bright, lively, and attractive 21-year-old. Open and direct in the interview, she was warmly appreciative of both her hospital treatment and also the outpatient psychotherapy that continued for 18 months following discharge. Betty described a period of some acting out immediately after discharge, which she had discussed openly with her psychotherapist and was able to resolve. After high school graduation, she worked in an antique shop for a year, then she enrolled in a local junior college. After a year, Betty transferred to a large university some distance away. At the time of the follow-up interview, Betty was a senior, was engaged to a young man with whom she had been living for approximately a year, and described her life in believably positive terms. Her fiance was a mature, hard-working young man. They had several close friends with whom they enjoyed many social activities.

Although Betty's parents had divorced following her hospital discharge, she remained close to both of them. She visited each frequently and indicated no further difficulties with them "once I got straightened out." Betty had worked part-time throughout her college years and she planned to continue working after graduation and marriage.

Although her behavior was somewhat erratic during the initial post-hospital year, Betty's course over the following five years appeared much more stable and mature. She was rated Good on all outcome scales, therefore Adaptive on the Global Level of Function.

The Follow-up Level of Function Scales, adapted from those used in other studies,[1,2,3] have proved to be useful measures for adolescent treatment outcome.

In addition, however, three other mental health professionals* also independently surveyed the same Follow-up Folders to record information on more specific characteristics such as marriages, divorces, number of children, living arrangements, details of academic and occupational performance, numbers and types of subsequent medical and psychiatric hospitalizations, specific legal difficulties, various patterns of drug and alcohol use and abuse, continuation of psychotherapy, rehospitalizations, and major remaining psychiatric symptomatology. None of the six raters were members of the Timberlawn Adolescent Service treatment team during the time these patients were in treatment.

RESULTS

On 15 of the 120 consecutive patients comprising the study group, the investigators were unable to obtain follow-up information sufficient to allow thorough judgments of outcome. These patients clearly were nonrepresentative of the overall group, a finding which merits

---

*Mark J. Blotcky, M.D., John C. Chelf, M. D., and Patsy K. Keyser, R.N., M.S.

further examination (see below). Three others had died, leaving 102 subjects for follow-up interviewing. For these 102 individuals (85 percent of the initial study group), the three judges of Level of Function at follow-up correlated strongly in their ratings, as shown in Table 6.

These reliability coefficients, all statistically significant, indicate substantial agreement among independent raters concerning the subjects' levels of functioning along these basic dimensions. Our data indicate clearly that independent reliable judgments concerning patients' adjustments on these critical outcome dimensions can be made.

Averaging the three outcome judgments (Table 7), the data illustrate the overall levels of functioning of the 105 former patients at the time of follow-up contact. (The three deceased patients, all apparent suicides, were arbitrarily given Poor ratings on all variables.)

Focusing upon the 105 rated cases, 28 (27 percent) were judged to be functioning at an essentially healthy global level of function, while 44 (42 percent) were described as Fair, and 33 (31 percent) were rated at a Poor level. If one follows the lead of previous studies in the field, combining Good and Fair outcome, and contrasts these with Poor outcome, 69 percent of the rated sample are evaluated as functioning at the higher level, with 31 percent at the lower level, an overall result that compares favorably with previous studies.

It is important to explore the characteristics of the patients from whom we were unable to obtain thorough follow-up information. It is noted above that the 15 former patients are not representative of the overall sample. This group differed primarily in severity of psychopathology, containing a disproportionate number of profoundly para-

TABLE 6

Interrater Reliability for Level of Function Scales*

Scale	Raters		
	A–B	A–C	B–C
Peer Relationships	.77	.77	.72
Family Relationships	.77	.74	.68
Occupational Functioning	.81	.79	.74
Global Level of Function	.79	.84	.76

*Pearson Product-Moment Correlation Coefficients. All coefficients are significant at $p < .001$ level.

TABLE 7

Level of Function Ratings*

Scale	n	Rating		
		% Good	% Fair	% Poor
Global Level	105	27	42	31
Peer Relationships	105	24	43	33
Family Relationships	105	17	49	34
Occupational Functioning	105	43	27	30

*Average of three raters' assessments.

noid, paranoid schizophrenic, and sociopathic youngsters (11 of 15). These syndromes also were noted with unusual frequency in their parents. Three of the 15 former patients refused to be interviewed, parents of three others refused our requests to interview their youngster, and in nine cases we were unable to locate any family member even with determined searching. Ten of these former patients were male, five were female.

Although we were unable to obtain sufficient information to allow thorough follow-up assessment for these 15 persons, we learned from a variety of informal sources of information that the majority were functioning at a level that would have been rated as Poor on the outcome dimensions (10 of the 15). The failure to locate or fully evaluate these individuals may tend, therefore, to bias our results in a positive direction.[5] While it is unlikely that all 15 of the unrated former patients would have been evaluated as Poor outcome, it is important to emphasize the need to keep attrition of subjects to a minimum if one is to derive accurate estimates of overall treatment effectiveness.

As noted above, three outcome evaluators examined the Follow-up Folders for information describing the former patients' current life adjustments. Two of the raters (PKK and JCC) independently abstracted case material in 18 content areas. Two raters were used for this task to assure that data would not be lost through oversight. The third rater, a child and adolescent psychiatrist (MJB), focused on the complex issues of post hospital drug and alcohol use and continuing psychiatric symptoms.

Approximately half of the follow-up group had continued to reside in the Dallas area, with the remainder located throughout the continental United States. At the time of the follow-up interview, about one-quarter of the group continued to live at home with their parents, another quarter with a spouse or lover, and the remainder lived either alone or with a friend. Less than half of the sample had married; of those who had married, half were divorced. Twenty-five of the group had one child, while three had two or more children.

Approximately three-quarters of the sample had graduated from high school at the time of the follow-up interview. Several were actively involved in college work, but only six had graduated from college. This is particularly notable since most of the study group came from middle- or upper-middle class, college-oriented families, and most were old enough to have been college graduates at the time of the follow-up interview. The severe educational deficits present at the time of hospital admission continued to exist for many of the former patients in spite of a very intensive focus upon educational achievement in the treatment program. On the other hand, many were pursuing college courses on a part-time basis, and it may well be that a substantial number will attain college degrees eventually.

In the vocational area, the majority of the subjects had some employment experience, but the average level of vocational function also was lower than one would expect to see in a nonpatient group of the same age and socioeconomic background. The majority of the group, however, were either actively involved in educational programs or were essentially self-supporting; a small number continued to require institutional care or economic support from their parents.

Despite a great deal of involvement by many in illegal activities before admission to the hospital, legal problems after discharge were rare or minor in nature. Improvements in this area were striking.

While about half of the group continued or returned to outpatient psychotherapy at some time during the follow-up interval, psychiatric rehospitalization occurred for about one-fifth of the subjects. Almost all of these rehospitalizations were for short intervals (a few days or weeks), generally occurring in the context of a crisis situation with rapid resolution.

About half of the patient group demonstrated some variety of troublesome behavior during the follow-up period; approximately one-fifth reported or demonstrated moderate-to-severe symptoms of depression during this period of time. Psychotic episodes were noted in 13 subjects during the follow-up years, and three of the group had committed suicide.

Almost all of the group used marijuana socially or experimentally at some time during the follow-up interval and most had used alcoholic beverages. About half of the group might be classified as drug or alcohol "abusers" at some time following hospital discharge, but the general pattern was for this abuse to occur in the first six to 18 months post-discharge, followed by a marked diminution in use. At the time of assessment, approximately 15 percent of the group might still be classified as alcohol or drug abusers. From one perspective, this is a large figure compared to the roughly 5 percent rate in the general population. From another perspective, the 15 percent rate is a substantial reduction from the 75 percent who had experienced some period of alcohol and/or drug abuse before hospitalization.

In summary, moderate-to-marked improvement in a variety of life areas is the modal expectation over the first three to eight years of post-hospital functioning for this group of young people, most of whom had failed to benefit from prior treatment. This ex-patient group demonstrated marked reductions (compared to prehospital functioning) in psychiatric symptomatology, drug and alcohol abuse, the need for psychotherapeutic treatment, problems with legal authorities, and an increase in their abilities to be self-supporting. Perhaps the least encouraging area at the time of follow-up was that of formal educational attainment; however, college experience more equivalent to their non-patient peers may still result for those attending college on an intermittent or part-time basis.

Our experience to date suggests that reliable and valid measures of treatment outcome are obtainable with practical follow-up procedures. This finding encourages the development of continued refinement in treatment assessment research.

REFERENCES

1. Garber, B. *Follow-up Study of Hospitalized Adolescents.* New York: Brunner/ Mazel, 1972.
2. Grob, M. C., & Singer, J. E. *Adolescent Patients in Transition: Impact and Out-*

come of Psychiatric Hospitalization. New York: Behavioral Publications, 1974.
3. Hartmann, E. H., Glasser, B. A., Greenblatt, M., Solomon, M. H., & Levinson, D. J. *Adolescents in a Mental Hospital.* New York: Grune & Stratton, 1968.
4. Lewis, J. M., Gossett, J. T., King, J. W., & Carson, D. I. Development of a pro-treatment group process among hospitalized adolescents. In S. C. Feinstein & P. L. Giovacchini (Eds.), *Adolescent Psychiatry: Developmental and Clinical Studies,* (Vol. 2). New York: Basic Books, 1973, pp. 351–362.
5. Penk, W. E., Uebersax, J. S., Charles, H. L., & Andrews, R. H. Psychological aspects of data loss in outcome research. *Evaluation Review,* 1981, *5,* 392–396.

CHAPTER 5

Descriptive Correlates of Treatment Outcome

In the last chapter we noted Adaptive (that is, Good or Fair) global outcome in 64-69 percent of the 120 former patients, with the difference between these two figures depending on assumptions one is willing to make concerning the outcome of the 15 former patients who were not interviewed. However, noting that two out of three discharged patients have shown significant improvement and are currently functioning reasonably well is merely the starting point for a more detailed examination of the characteristics of those with different outcome results.

This chapter will examine a variety of characteristics to obtain a clearer picture at admission and at five-year follow-up of those patients judged to have an Adaptive overall level of functioning versus those judged to have a Poor level of function at follow-up.

HOSPITAL ADMISSION INFORMATION

Gender

In this, as in all subsequent comparisons in this chapter, we will combine Good and Fair global outcome and will exclude the 15 former patients who were not interviewed at follow-up.

TABLE 8

Characteristics of Those with Adaptive and Poor Levels of Function at Follow-Up

Characteristics	n	Level of Function	
		Adaptive	Poor
Gender			
Male	58	37	21
Female	47	35	12
	$X^2 = .92, p = $ n.s.		
Age at Admission			
13–15	38	27	11
16	21	14	7
17	31	22	9
18–19	15	9	6
	$X^2 = .73, p = $ n.s.		
Intelligence Quotient			
≤ 89	4	1	3
90–109	26	19	7
110–119	27	18	9
120–129	28	20	8
≥ 130	17	13	4
	$X^2 = 4.6, p = $ n.s.		
Diagnosis			
Neurotic Disorders	9	7	2
Personality Disorders	71	53	18
Psychotic Disorders	25	12	13
	$X^2 = 6.35, p < .025$		
Previous Treatment			
None	6	4	2
Outpatient Only	50	37	13
Outpatient and In-patient	49	31	18
(Prior Inpatient 1x	26	19	7)
(Prior Inpatient 2–4x	23	12	11)
	$X^2 = 1.32, p = $ n.s.		
Months of Hospital Stay			
≤ 3	15	8	7
4–11	24	15	9
12–18	29	23	6
19–24	24	17	7
≥ 25	13	9	4
	$X^2 = 3.67, p = $ n.s.		

68

TABLE 8 *(continued)*

| Characteristics | n | Level of Function | |
		Adaptive	Poor
Type of Discharge			
Treatment Refused	6	5	1
Transferred	9	2	7
Treatment Incom-			
plete	55	34	21
Treatment Com-			
pleted	35	31	4
	$X^2 = 17.4, p < .001$		

Results in Table 8 indicate 74 percent Adaptive outcome for the females, with a 64 percent Adaptive outcome for the males. While not statistically significant, this finding is consistent with clinical differences noted between our male and female patient populations. It is our impression that in this sample adolescent males are more severely disturbed on the average at admission than are adolescent females. This may reflect greater parental and social tolerance for disturbed behavior among adolescent males before hospitalization. Staff ratings of severity of psychopathology at the time of admission indicate some support for this clinical impression (Table 9).*

TABLE 9

Gender Difference in Gossett-
Timberlawn Adolescent
Psychopathology Scale Scores

| | Difference of Means | |
	Male	Female
N	51	34
$\overline{X}$	141.37	126.76
SD	14.79	19.88

$t = 3.66$ with 57 degrees of freedom $p < .01$

---

*The Gossett-Timberlawn Adolescent Psychopathology Scale assesses patients' current level of functioning along 10 dimensions and yields scores ranging from 10 to 190 with increasing scores reflecting greater psychopathology. The Scale is described in Chapter 6 and is reproduced in Appendix A.

In addition, it is our clinical impression that in an insight oriented, relationship based, long-term treatment program, adolescent males present (on the average) somewhat deeper and more prolonged treatment resistances. Another impression is that there may be greater social pressures for academic and vocational achievement with less social tolerance for overt economic and emotional dependency in young adult men as compared to young adult women. This may create somewhat higher outcome level of function demands for young men at follow-up.

Age at Admission

The majority of patients were 15 to 17 at the time of admission, with a small number being slightly younger or older. Virtually identical long-term outcome for each age group demonstrates the lack of relationship between admission age and outcome (Table 8).

Intelligence

At the time of admission, each patient was given an intellectual evaluation using the Shipley-Hartford Intelligence Test. A small number who presented particular problems relating to intellectual capabilities were subsequently given a Wechsler Intelligence Scale for Children or a Wechsler Adult Intelligence Scale. Information presented in Table 8 is based upon the initial Shipley-Hartford Intelligence Test.

Three individuals could not be evaluated with this instrument during the initial weeks of hospitalization. For the remaining 102, the figures suggest that above an I.Q. level of 90 tested intelligence did not relate to outcome. However, in the very small subgroup of below-average intelligence, only one of the four individuals had a Fair outcome. Although the numbers are small, this suggests that disturbed youngsters with below-average intellectual abilities may have an unusually difficult task overcoming both intellectual limitations and severe psychopathology (see Chapter 2).

Psychiatric Diagnosis

The first several weeks of each patient's hospital stay were devoted to a thorough clinical evaluation, including multiple patient and family interviews, psychological testing, and a two-hour intake staffing drawing together the results of observations by team psychiatrists, psychologists, social workers, nurses, teachers, psychiatric aides, and activities therapists. During or following this staffing, the administrative psychiatrist, in consultation with other team members, would derive a detailed case formulation and treatment recommendations. One part of the case formulation was the derivation of an official (DSM-II) diagnosis.

Collapsing these diagnoses into neurotic, personality disorder, and psychotic, the results given in Table 8 were obtained.

. Although percentages must be viewed tentatively when based upon small numbers, it is striking to note Adaptive outcome with 78 percent of the patients experiencing severe neurotic disorders, a similar 75 percent Adaptive outcome among the personality disorders, but only 48 percent Adaptive outcome among the youngsters with psychotic diagnoses. Within the three major categories of neurotic, personality, and psychotic disorders, similarities between specific diagnoses were more striking than were the differences, with the exception that the generally positive outcome for the personality disorder group was not found for those youngsters with an antisocial diagnosis; in this small subgroup, the majority have not done well.

Previous Psychological Treatment

Ninety-four percent of the patient group had one or more unsuccessful treatment experiences before being hospitalized at Timberlawn.

Of the six youngsters who came to Timberlawn without previous treatment, four were doing well at follow-up. Approximately half of the patient group had received one or more attempts at outpatient psychotherapy prior to the index hospitalization, with the remaining half of the group having been hospitalized one or more times before coming to Timberlawn.

The data in Table 8 demonstrate that type and number of previous treatment attempts did not relate significantly to overall outcome.

HOSPITAL LENGTH OF STAY AND TREATMENT COMPLETION

Duration of Treatment

Problems in using hospital length of stay as a measurement of treatment success are discussed in detail in Chapter 10.

In a long-term treatment program, discharges taking place in the first three months usually involve parental inability or refusal to follow treatment recommendations. Among this group of 15 patients (five of whom later received further inpatient care elsewhere), half had Adaptive outcomes, and half had Poor outcomes. Among the remaining 90 patients who stayed in the treatment program for longer periods of time, approximately 70 percent showed Adaptive outcome. The data suggest that the optimal treatment range for the majority of the patients admitted to the program was 12–24 months.

Completion of Inpatient Treatment

Following the initial several weeks of intensive evaluation of their adolescent, six families rejected the staff's treatment recommendations and withdrew their youngster from the program. At follow-up, five of these former patients were evaluated as doing well. While at first glance this might suggest the parents may have been wise to refuse recommendations for inpatient care, it should be noted that two of the six subsequently were hospitalized elsewhere for lengthy inpatient treatment programs, and all five of the successful outcome cases subsequently received effective additional treatment.

Nine adolescents were transferred from the Timberlawn treatment program to other institutions following unsuccessful attempts of varying periods of time to treat them in this setting. Only two of those youngsters were functioning at even a Fair level at follow-up, while about two-thirds of the individuals who accomplished some goals but were discharged prematurely were found to be functioning well at follow-up.

POST-DISCHARGE INFORMATION

Type of Follow-up Interview

Face-to-face interviews with former patients were obtained with approximately half of the overall group. Generally, these were young men and women who lived in or near Dallas; however, several former patients traveled long distances for personal interviews. More commonly, former patients living some distance from Dallas were interviewed by telephone. Almost identical percentages of young people were rated Good, Fair, and Poor, whether they were interviewed in person or by telephone, and it was the strong impression of the interviewer (JTG) that telephone contacts provide excellent quality data for follow-up assessment if the interviewer is known to the ex-patients.

Parents of former patients more often preferred to be interviewed by telephone, with a small group willing to come to the Foundation for a personal interview (parents from 13 families), and another small group requesting interviews at their home or office (parents from 16 families). Again, there appeared to be no relationship between the rated level of function of the former patient and the location or type of interview. The parents' interviewer (FDB) was impressed also with the sense of thoroughness, completeness, and experienced validity of the telephone follow-up interviews.

Follow-up Interval

The Pilot Studies described in Chapter 3 demonstrated relative behavioral instability for many of the patients during their first year after discharge. Conducting follow-up interviews one to three years after discharge, however, revealed 78 percent Adaptive outcome in the Main Study (Table 10). Among the group of youngsters seen four or five years after discharge, 69 percent were doing well, while 65 percent

TABLE 10

Characteristics Post-discharge of Those with Adaptive and Poor Levels of Function at Follow-up

Characteristics	n	Level of Function	
		Adaptive	Poor
Interval Until Follow-up			
1–3 Years	18	14	4
4–5 Years	35	24	11
≥ 6 Years	52	34	18
$X^2 = 1.0, p = $ n.s.			
Educational Attainment			
High School Drop-out	23	10	13
GED	26	18	8
High School Diploma	50	43	7
$X^2 = 14.1, p < .001$			
No College	42	21	21
Currently in College	56	46	10
College Graduate	3	2	1
Currently in Graduate School	3	3	0
$X^2 = 12.99, p < .005$			
Employment			
Employed	66	54	12
Unemployed	35	18	17
$X^2 = 8.89, p < .005$			
Marital Status			
Married	19	17	2
Separated or Divorced	21	14	7
Never Married	65	41	24
$X^2 = 4.86, p < .05$			
Living Arrangement			
Alone	23	13	10
In Institution	3	0	3
With Others			
Parents	28	21	7
Spouse	19	17	2
Lover	12	8	4
Roomate	16	13	3
$X^2 = 13.69, p < .01$			

74

TABLE 10 (*continued*)

| Characteristics | n | Level of Function | |
		Adaptive	Poor
Medical Hospitaliza-tion			
None	54	40	14
1	30	23	7
2	9	7	2
≥3	10	2	8
	$X^2 = 13.3, p < .005$		
Psychotherapy After Discharge			
Continued as Recommended	47	38	9
Continued Briefly	25	15	10
Discontinued at Discharge	33	19	14
	$X^2 = 5.95, p < .05$		
Legal Difficulties			
None	66	50	16
1 Offense	21	17	4
≥2 Offenses	18	5	13
	$X^2 = 16.73, p < .001$		
Use of Marijuana			
Never Used	10	6	4
Used at Some Time	95	66	29
	$X^2 = .07, p = $ n.s.		
Current Marijuana Use			
None	31	24	7
Social	45	37	8
Abuse	15	3	12
	$X^2 = 21.7, p < .005$		

of those interviewed six or more years after discharge were doing well. These differences, although modest, are misleading, however, in that the group of 52 youngsters interviewed six to eight years after discharge contained a disproportionate number of individuals who were unusually hard to locate, which in turn biased that group toward more severe psychopathology. The procedure of contacting former patients began in the order of their hospital discharge, but those who could not be located initially tended to accumulate, concurrently building up post-discharge time. When finally located, these more mobile persons did tend to have shown deeper characterological problems at admission and during treatment. This biasing effect of severity of psychopathology on ease of locating (and, therefore, indirectly on length of follow-up interval) should always be considered in comparing such groups.

Educational Status*

As indicated in Table 10, the majority of high school dropouts were not functioning well at follow-up.

All of the former patients were old enough at the time of follow-up to have attended college if they so desired. Approximately 60 percent of the group had enrolled for college work at the time of follow-up, a finding which reflects the basically middle- and upper-middle class orientation of the group. Within the very small group that had graduated from college at the time of follow-up, five out of six were doing well as compared to a 50–50 outcome attainment for the group that had not attended college.

Occupational Status

All of the former patients were also old enough at the time of follow-up to be working. Of those who were employed, the majority were doing well in other respects also, whereas among the unemployed, outcome was much more evenly divided with approximately half functioning poorly.

It is of special interest that it is within the area of employment that former psychiatric patients appear to have the greatest difficulty. Anthony, Buell, Sharratt, and Althoff[1] in their excellent review article

---

*Educational status and the additional items under Post-discharge Information were considered by the outcome judges in deriving their Follow-up Level of Function ratings; therefore, significant relationships are not unexpected.

found, for example, that it is relatively easy to bring about improvement in psychiatric patients' symptomatic functioning while the patients are still in the hospital setting and that improved interpersonal relating transfers much better to post-discharge settings than does the ability to obtain and hold employment. Summarizing the results of a number of studies, Anthony et al. found that during the year following hospital discharge, only 20–30 percent of former patients engage in full-time academic or vocational pursuits. This figure apparently remains fairly constant, as they also reviewed another study demonstrating 25 percent full-time employment three years post-discharge for another group of former patients. Viewed from the perspective of that baseline, the current finding that 65 percent of the former patients in this group were employed three to eight years post-discharge is encouraging.

Marital Status

Of the 19 patients married at the time of follow-up interview, almost all (17) were doing well.

Two-thirds of the separated and divorced former patients were functioning at an Adaptive level, with a slightly lower percentage of those never married also functioning at an Adaptive level. With an average age in the early to mid-twenties, it is probably too early for failure to marry to be a powerful predictor of poor long-term outcome.

Living Arrangement

Three former patients were institutionalized at the time of follow-up. Of the 23 former patients living alone, slightly over half were doing well; the majority of the former patients, however, were living in some variety of more or less close relationship; that is, with a lover, with parents, with a roommate, or with a spouse. Table 10 depicts those living arrangements.

Those able to maintain a social living arrangement appear to have a better chance of overall adequate functioning.

Physical Health

In general, this was a physically healthy group of young people. Keeping in mind that almost all former patients were between the ages of 20 and 25 at the time of follow-up, it is not surprising that few had experienced serious physical difficulties. The small number of serious physical illnesses or accidents that had resulted in hospitalization, however, did tend to relate to Poor psychiatric status, as seen in Table 10. The majority of the young people in this sample had not experienced any serious physical problems during the follow-up period, nor had they required unusual medical treatment or hospitalization for physical illnesses or accidents. However, a small subgroup (10 patients) had experienced three or more hospitalizations for physical illness or accident since discharge, and among these 10 patients, eight had Poor psychiatric outcomes. Among the five young women in this group (four Poor and one Adaptive outcome), each had one or more abortions or deliveries, although only one had ever married; two of the women had been hospitalized following physical fights with boyfriends, and two were hospitalized as a result of serious injuries sustained in automobile accidents.

Among the five young men (four Poor and one Adaptive outcome), three had experienced multiple hospitalizations due to drug overdose or drug-related hepatitis, one experienced multiple hospitalizations related to an epileptic condition, and one had experienced a series of physical illnesses which represented a continuation of psychosomatic problems very much in evidence before the index psychiatric hospitalization.

Continuation of Psychotherapy

Continuation of individual psychotherapy was recommended for all patients at the time of discharge. Table 10 details the outcome of those recommendations.

Of those who continued in psychotherapy until a mutually agreed upon termination (or for at least one year post-discharge), 38 of 47 were doing well at follow-up. Additionally, 25 youngsters saw their therapist a few times after discharge, but terminated before the therapist felt was best. A lesser percentage of this group was doing well at follow-up. Among the 33 adolescents who terminated psychotherapy at the time of discharge, almost half were functioning at a Poor level at follow-up.

A review of hospital recidivism[1] indicates an average 70 percent rehospitalization rate five years post-discharge for patients from a variety of psychiatric hospitals. In this group of 105 young people, 20 had been rehospitalized by the time of the follow-up interview, although only two of that 20 were hospitalized at the time of follow-up. This 19 percent rehospitalization rate compares favorably with the 70 percent rate noted in the literature.

Of these 20 youngsters, almost all had been treated in Timberlawn for several months or more, but very few had been discharged as having completed their inpatient treatment program.

The largest group of rehospitalized youngsters included five boys and two girls (all given personality disorder diagnoses at Timberlawn) noted to be seriously depressed during hospital treatment at Timberlawn and whose depressive symptoms continued and worsened in late adolescence or young adulthood. Each of these seven individuals was later hospitalized following serious suicide attempts; two subsequently committed suicide.

Another group of six former patients (five female and one male) were later rehospitalized with schizophrenic reactions; three had well-established schizophrenic syndromes before and during their Timberlawn treatment, while the remainder were diagnosed as severe personality disorders as adolescents.

Another group of four young men given sociopathic diagnoses at Timberlawn were later rehospitalized; two continued with antisocial behavior, while two later developed classical paranoid schizophrenic syndromes as young adults. One of these ex-patients committed suicide.

Finally, the remaining three former patients (two males and one female) were subsequently hospitalized with clear-cut manic episodes, although all three had been diagnosed as personality disorders during adolescence. Although in retrospect one can identify periods of hyper-activity, verbal overproductiveness, labile moods, marked irritability, and nonpsychotic grandiosity in all three of these youngsters, those characteristics did not at the time appear significantly different from similar behaviors and symptoms seen in many other adolescent personality disorder patients.

Legal Problems

The majority of the group (66 former patients) had no encounters with the law following discharge. Twenty-one former patients had been arrested for one offense since discharge, but 17 of these individuals were functioning well at follow-up. Of the 21 offenses, 11 involved traffic or misdemeanor problems, while only one was a violent felony. The remaining nine legal difficulties all involved arrests for possession of illegal drugs. In each of these latter cases, the arrest and subsequent proceedings markedly discouraged continued illicit drug involvement, and all nine of these young adults were included in the Adaptive outcome category.

However, of the subgroup of 18 multiple offenders (two or more traffic, drug, other misdemeanors, or felony arrests), most were not functioning well at follow-up. Considering the frequency of illegal activities in which this patient group was involved before long-term treatment, it is quite striking that only 18 (17 percent) of the group were multiple offenders following discharge.

Drug and Alcohol Abuse

When asked about drug and alcohol use, 95 of the 105 former patients indicated they had smoked marijuana, while only 10 denied any experience with this drug. Whether they had or had not smoked marijuana did not appear to relate to long-term outcome.

When asked to describe their marijuana usage in more detail, however, it was usually possible to categorize such usage as social (occasional marijuana use that did not appear to interfere with vocational, interpersonal, or mental status functioning) versus abuse (drug use which did appear to be involved in some interpersonal, vocational, or mental status impairment).

The majority of the 31 patients who indicated that they were no longer smoking marijuana were doing well. Most of the 45 social marijuana users also were doing well; however, for the youngsters who acknowledged usage to the point that it did interfere in some significant aspect in their life, drug involvement was part of a pattern of Poor overall functioning. These 15 subjects were involved in more-or-less heavy drinking and usage of other drugs, as well, in contrast to the social marijuana smokers and the nonsmokers, most of whom either did not drink or were social drinkers; none of the social marijuana smokers were frequent users of other drugs.

Approximately three-quarters of this study group were heavy users or abusers of a variety of illicit drugs before hospitalization. Following discharge, approximately half were involved in experimental or social use of hallucinogens, stimulants, depressants, or other "street" drugs. However, within a few months following discharge, almost all had restricted their drug usage to social or recreational reliance upon alcohol and marijuana. A small subgroup (10–15 former patients) had continued moderate to heavy involvement in illicit drug use more or less continuously during the follow-up years. Such continued heavy usage through late adolescence and into young adulthood, while rare, was quite ominous in that it invariably was correlated with Poor functioning in all significant life areas.

It should be noted that this small group of chronic polydrug abusers were also almost without exception heavy drinkers. There were an additional three or four heavy drinkers (alcoholics or pre-alcoholics) who were not heavy drug users. Striking in the histories of the continued chronic heavy drug abusers was their gradual shift through adolescence and into adulthood away from more or less exclusive reliance on drugs (with heated philosophical objections to the use of alcohol), into increasing reliance upon alcohol and a diminution of defensive philosophizing about the benefits of drug involvement. The majority of these youngsters appeared in their early and mid-twenties to be well on the way to chronic, severe alcoholism and, in that respect, looked quite similar to young alcoholics in the years before the so-called "psychedelic" drug revolution of the late 1960s and the 1970s.

Deaths

At the time of follow-up (five years post-discharge), there had been four deaths in the group of 105 former patients. All four deceased former patients were male, all had originally received personality disorder diagnoses (although one subsequently developed a paranoid schizophrenic syndrome in addition to antisocial behaviors) and three were clearly intentional suicides. Combining these four deaths with several others known to the investigators from the earlier Pilot Study group and several that have occurred in youngsters treated in the same program subsequent to the research study group, it appears that a relatively constant rate of about one former inpatient has died each year, with most being clearly intentional suicides. Since the program discharges about 20-25 patients a year, the annual death rate is about four or five percent.

Clinicians have long been aware of the dangerously self-destructive potential of severely depressed individuals and certain schizophrenics. However, it is striking that in this population of adolescents, the majority of whom exhibit (nonpsychotic) severe impulse-ridden personality disorders upon admission, late adolescent or young adult suicide is a very real possibility. The internal suffering and desperation of such individuals may often be obscured by the troublesomeness of their behavior to others. Our data suggest that the clinician should remain sensitive to this internal distress, particularly in young, male, severe personality disorder patients.

Other Severe Psychiatric Disturbance

Thirteen of the 105 former patients appeared by history to have experienced some variety of diagnosable psychotic reaction subsequent to discharge. Ten of these patients were functioning at a Poor level at follow-up. Similarly, 10 former patients appeared to have experienced serious episodes of paranoid symptoms since discharge, and eight of these 10 were functioning at a Poor level at follow-up. On a more positive note, 19 of the former patients had experienced serious depressive episodes during the follow-up interval, but almost all (17) of this group were functioning at an Adaptive level at follow-up; thus, it appears that serious depression is a relatively common occurrence for this group of young people, but it is seldom chronically incapacitating.

Nearly half of the total group (49 out of 105) were rated as having been involved in some variety of "acting out" after hospital discharge. Generally, this involved a return to some prior behavioral difficulties in the initial months post-discharge. This regressive period often lasted six to 12 months, but rarely continued beyond 18 months post-discharge for those subsequently able to attain Adaptive outcome. Of this group of 49 youngsters, more than half (27) were functioning well at follow-up.

SUMMARY

It appears that of every 100 patients discharged, about 50 will function well from time of discharge through a five-year follow-up interval, although occasional periods of depression will occur for some. The remaining 50 youngsters will leave the treatment program either not functioning well at the time of discharge or will regress to a variety of acting-out behaviors following discharge. Within this group of 50, about 20-25 can be expected to show marked improvement after six to 18 months. Most of the remaining (25-30) will still be doing very poorly five or more years after discharge, and this will be reflected in drug and/or alcohol abuse, antisocial acting out, psychotic episodes, alienation from family and friends, and failures at school and vocation, with rehospitalizations or legal incarcerations. Several of this latter group may die during this interval.

The focus on negative outcomes, however, should not obscure the fact that about 65-70 percent of the original group will show substantial treatment benefits, reflected in markedly improved peer and family relationships, more successful educational and vocational functioning, reduced symptomatic status, and much greater subjective contentment. The fact that this result has occurred with a group of youngsters almost all of whom were failures from prior outpatient and/or inpatient treatment is, in our judgment, most encouraging.

Although the predictive power of severity and chronicity of present-ing psychopathology has been reconfirmed, completion of the goals of the inpatient phase of treatment and continuation of psychotherapy after discharge remain cornerstones of effective intervention.

REFERENCE

1. Anthony, W. A., Buell, G. J., Sharratt, S., & Althoff, M. E. Efficacy of psychia-tric rehabilitation. *Psychological Bulletin,* 1972, *78,* 447–456.

CHAPTER 6

Clinical Scale Correlates of Outcome

Early in the evolution of the Adolescent Treatment Assessment Project, the need for measuring instruments of treatment and outcome variables was clear. Review of the literature (Chapter 2) supported the need for such instruments. Severity of individual psychopathology, chronicity of symptoms, and the level of function of the family of origin were identified as powerful treatment and outcome determinants for which adequate measuring instruments appropriate to adolescent inpatients and their families were not available. During the time these scales were being developed, the research literature suggested that "locus of control" also might be useful for treatment outcome prediction.

This chapter concerns findings that correlate with level of function at outcome: severity of psychopathology, chronicity of symptoms, family level of competence, and locus of control.

SEVERITY OF PSYCHOPATHOLOGY

Prior outcome studies indicate that the severity of psychopathology at the time of a patient's admission to a hospital is the strongest predictor of long-term outcome (Chapter 2). This finding is reported repeatedly, despite common reliance upon a simple measure of severity of psychopathology which uses the broad diagnostic categories of neurosis, personality disorder, and psychosis. We were unable to locate a refined instrument to assess severity of adolescent psychopathology suitable for both clinical and research purposes.

Luborsky, however, reports a promising instrument for the assessment of severity of psychopathology in adults.[7] This instrument (the Health-Sickness Rating Scale) provides a single global dimension upon which patients could be assigned a score ranging from 100 ("an ideal state of complete functioning integration") to 0 ("any condition which, if unattended, would quickly result in the patient's death"). Several scale points between these extremes were defined, with accompanying clinical examples.

In applying the Luborsky Health-Sickness Rating Scale to several adolescent patients, it appeared that the instrument could be made more sensitive to adolescent developmental issues. By modifying it to include those issues and to make it more specific, the Gossett-Timberlawn Adolescent Psychopathology Scale* was developed. It consists of 10 clinical subscales:

1) *Autonomy*—the person's ability to function independently versus the need to be protected and/or supported by a therapist or a hospital.
2) *Diagnostic Severity*—the degree of personality integration or disorganization in psychodiagnostic terms.
3) *Subjective Discomfort*—the degree of distress consciously experienced by the individual while engaged in age-appropriate scholastic, vocational, and interpersonal situations.
4) *Environmental Effect*—the manner in which the person's behavior influences those around him or her.
5) *School Performance*—level of academic achievement in relation to ability level.
6) *Interests*—breadth and depth of interests.
7) *Intimacy of Relationships*—qualities of interpersonal warmth, intimacy, and genuineness.
8) *Maturity of Object Relationships*—the nature of the person's most meaningful relationship ties.

---

*Appendix A

9) *Insight*—the degree to which the person's perception of his or her disturbance corresponds to assessment made by others.

10) *Motivation*—the amount of goal-directed energy the person can expend toward realistic self-exploration and productive personality change.

Each of the subscales contains 10 defined levels of severity, ranging from very healthy to very disturbed, and intermediate rating points create 19-point subscales. A patient may receive a score of 1 to 19 on each subscale, and thus could obtain a total Psychopathology Score ranging from 10 (maximum health) to 190 (maximum dysfunction). Additional features of the Scale include a section for the rater to evaluate the degree of familiarity with the adolescent patient and how well the rater liked the subject.

By the time the final form of the scale was developed, a number of the 120 youngsters in the Main Study group were beyond the point of initial evaluation. The final form of the scale, however, was used on 71 consecutive patients immediately following their initial weeks of inpatient evaluation. Clinical staff present at the intake evaluation conference completed the scale independently for each youngster. The number of raters assessing individual patients range from two to 18, with a mean of 11 raters per patient.

Not all clinical staff were present at every intake evaluation conference. The Adolescent Service Director,* the Director of the Boys' Unit,** and the senior author (JTG), however, were present at a majority.

Interrater reliability data for the three raters on 49 subjects are presented in Table 11.

The median interrater correlation for the total Adolescent Psychopathology Scale score was .84. The various subscale reliabilities also appear adequate, especially considering the clinical complexity of the rating task.

After adequate scale reliabilities are established, it is important to

---

*Joe W. King, M.D.
**Doyle I. Carson, M.D.

Interrater Reliability on the Gossett-Timberlawn Adolescent Psychopathology Scale*

Subscale	Raters		
	A–B	A–C	B–C
Autonomy	.70	.62	.73
Diagnostic Severity	.68	.74	.64
Subjective Discomfort	.62	.52	.62
Environmental Effect	.34	.59	.51
School Performance	.89	.91	.88
Interests	.73	.49	.42
Intimacy of Relationships	.52	.48	.45
Maturity of Relationships	.54	.53	.65
Insight	.50	.45	.66
Motivation	.72	.62	.65
Total Scale Score	.84	.81	.86

*Pearson Product Moment Correlation Coefficients, $p < .01$
$N = 49$

determine the relationships between an instrument's subscales. In general, one hopes to find that all subscales are contributing meaningfully to the total score, but that no two or more subscales are correlated so highly with each other as to be redundant. Subscale intercorrelations are presented in Table 12. The figures suggest that each of the subscales contributes to the total scale score in a positive and meaningful fashion. The highest subscale intercorrelation is that between the measures of Insight and Motivation ($r = .80$). This level of correlation suggests these dimensions are similar, but is low enough to leave room for each subscale to offer a unique contribution to the total score.

The two subscales revealing highest correlations with the total Psychopathology score are each general measures of overall level of competence (Autonomy and Diagnostic Severity). The similarity of these two subscales to the Endicott-Spitzer Global Assessment Scale is striking.[3] The Gossett-Timberlawn Adolescent Psychopathology Scale and the Endicott-Spitzer Global Assessment Scale were developed independently during the same time period, and both use Luborsky's Health-Sickness Scale as a starting point. Their common origins and the similar goals sought by the researchers probably account for the similarities in form and content.

In addition to the excellent predictive power of the Adolescent Psychopathology Scale (see Table 13), the subscale scores yield a patient profile revealing important areas of strength and dysfunction with clear treatment implications.

Using total scores of 135 or less and 136 or more and predicting Adaptive outcome for the low scores (less psychopathology) and Poor outcome for the higher scores (greater psychopathology), correct outcome predictions are made for 46 of the 71 patients (65 percent). Comparable results can be attained by using either the Diagnostic Severity or Environmental Effect subscales only, although they yield less even-

TABLE 12

Intercorrelations of the Subscales of the Gossett-Timberlawn Adolescent Psychopathology Scale*

Subscale	(1)	(2)	(3)	(4)	(5)	(6)	(7)	(8)	(9)	(10)	(11)
(1) Autonomy		.77	.50	.72	.51	.61	.63	.65	.71	.73	.88
(2) Diagnostic Severity			.69	.67	.47	.53	.65	.70	.67	.66	.84
(3) Subjective Discomfort				.45	.35	.33	.45	.54	.41	.31	.60
(4) Environmental Effect					.31	.42	.48	.52	.53	.47	.68
(5) School Performance						.41	.49	.43	.44	.41	.68
(6) Interests							.52	.56	.56	.65	.72
(7) Intimacy of Relationships								.61	.59	.60	.71
(8) Maturity of Relationships									.63	.51	.76
(9) Insight										.80	.81
(10) Motivation											.82
(11) Total Scale Score											—

*Pearson Product Moment Correlation Coefficients
N = 71

TABLE 13

Contingency Table of Gossett-Timberlawn Adolescent Psychopathology Subscales and Level of Function Scale

Score	n	Outcome	
		Adaptive	Poor
Autonomy			
≤ 14	36	29	7
≥ 15	35	20	15
	$X^2 = 3.5, p < .05$		
Diagnostic Severity			
≤ 14	40	32	8
≥ 15	31	17	14
	$X^2 = 3.8, p < .025$		
Subjective Discomfort			
≤ 14	34	28	6
≥ 15	37	21	16
	$X^2 = 4.3, p < .025$		
Environmental Effect			
≤ 13	40	33	7
≥ 14	31	16	15
	$X^2 = 6.4, p < .01$		
School Performance			
≤ 12	28	25	3
≥ 13	43	24	19
	$X^2 = 7.4, p < .005$		
Interests			
≤ 16	36	29	7
≥ 17	35	20	15
	$X^2 = 3.5, p < .05$		
Intimacy of Relationships			
≤ 13	27	20	7
≥ 14	44	29	15
	$X^2 = .21, p = $ n.s.		
Maturity of Relationships			
≤ 12	36	29	7
≥ 13	35	20	15
	$X^2 = 3.5, p < .05$		

TABLE 13 (*continued*)

Score	n	Outcome	
		Adaptive	Poor
Insight			
≤ 14	31	25	6
≥ 15	40	24	16
	$X^2 = 2.6, p = $ n.s.		
Motivation			
≤ 14	36	28	8
≥ 15	35	21	14
	$X^2 = 1.9, p = $ n.s.		
Total Scale Score			
≤ 135	32	28	4
≥ 136	39	21	18
	$X^2 = 7.8, p < .005$		

ly distributed outcome predictions; that is, while they appear to be as good or slightly better than the total score at predicting Adaptive outcome, they were not as accurate as the total score for the prediction of Poor outcome. The combination of high interrater reliability, strong correlation with outcome, and impressive ability to identify Adaptive versus Poor outcome cases suggests that Diagnostic Severity is the most predictive subscale.

ONSET OF SYMPTOMATOLOGY

Review of follow-up studies of adolescent inpatient treatment (Chapter 2) suggests that a group of 13 characteristics might differentiate more recent, stress-related symptomatic pictures from those of a more chronic nature with insidious development. An initial screening of hospital records for report of the 13 characteristics in a group of 50 adolescents discharged from Timberlawn between August 1966 and June 1968 was conducted. This search reveals that the following six of the 13 variables do not relate meaningfully to the long-term outcome information that had already been collected for this sample of patients (Chapter 3):

1) *Psychopathology in Siblings.* The individual with a chronic disorder is presumed more likely to have disturbed siblings than is an individual with a more acute disorder. The case histories examined, however, so rarely include scoreable information about the psychological health or pathology of the patient's siblings that this factor cannot be evaluated.

2) *Heterosexual Experiences.* The presence or absence of intimate heterosexual experience appears to be a highly predictive prognostic factor for adult psychotic patients, but this variable does not appear to relate significantly to outcome for patients ages 13-17 with a wide variety of psychiatric disturbance. Information on sexual experience frequently is not included in the hospital records; when it is, however, the patient's statements to different staff members are frequently contradictory, and the versions given by patients and by their parents are often at odds.

3) *Rate of Symptom Onset.* Evaluating gradual versus sudden onset of disabling symptoms from the hospital charts proved fruitless. This variable may be relevant in the small number of cases of severe psychosis, but appears to have little usefulness for the wider range of early developing borderline and other personality disorders more often seen in the hospital.

4) *Intensity of Symptom Onset.* Almost every adolescent admitted to a psychiatric hospital has experienced "stormy" functioning immediately prior to admission; thus, a suicide attempt, marked depression, running away, sexual acting out, illicit drug usage, marked school failure, or family turmoil immediately prior to admission are so common that they do not differentiate Adaptive from Poor outcome.

5) *Precipitating Stresses.* Examination of the events immediately preceding hospitalization almost invariably produces evidence for "understandable" or "believable" stress; therefore, this factor also had no predictive power.

6) *Rate of Symptomatic Change Early in Hospitalization.* This may be a powerful predictor, but the hospital case records of these subjects do not yield sufficient details about symptomatic change during the initial weeks of hospitalization to allow a rating on this variable to be accomplished.

After eliminating these six of the 13 factors suggested in the literature, measures were constructed for the remaining seven factors based upon the information obtained from the case histories. The result is the Onset of Symptomatology Scale,* which measures seven variables that can be evaluated from a hospital case history. The subscales are labeled: 1) Psychological Trauma; 2) Physical Trauma; 3) Behavior Control; 4) Academic Progress; 5) Peer Relationships; 6) Passivity-Aggressiveness Deviance; and 7) Symptom Duration. Each is rated on a continuum from 0 to 4 in the direction of increasing psychopathology. The total scores from the subscales may vary from 0 to 28. Low scores reflect syndromes of a reactive nature and high scores indicate a process disturbance.

To test the usefulness of the scale, ratings for each of the patients in the Pilot Study (Chapter 3) were made both by the scale developer (JTG) and by an experienced child and adolescent psychiatrist functioning outside the hospital setting who was unfamiliar with either the hospital treatment or the follow-up status of the patient sample.**

The total Onset of Symptomatology Scale scores of the two judges have a linear correlation coefficient of .79, $p < .001$. The Onset of Symptomatology Scale score related significantly to independently derived level of function at follow-up ratings. Examination of the relationship of the ratings to follow-up indicates that the Scale is most discriminating at the reactive end; that is, youngsters arriving at the hospital with indication of a recent onset disorder almost invariably are doing well at follow-up.

Those who present at the time of admission with process-oriented life histories, however, appear to have a 50-50 likelihood of functioning well several years after hospital treatment. This finding is consistent with that of earlier studies which suggest that a generally "healthy" early history provides a substantial bulwark against later life stress, while disturbed or even bizarre early life histories do not necessarily predict serious life-long disturbances.[10,11] Many individuals

---

*Appendix B
**John E. Meeks, M.D.

whose early life histories are as seriously disturbed as those of many hospital inpatients function well in society. In addition, the results are consistent with clinical observations that intensive, long-term psychiatric treatment can benefit not only those with reactive disturbances, but in a significant number of cases, those with process disturbances as well.

Inasmuch as the predictive power of the scale was measured (in the Pilot Study) using substantially the same group of patients whose case histories had led to the development of the scale items themselves, cross-validation was in order. That is, the scale needed to be applied to a completely new sample with new judges to see if it continued to relate meaningfully to long-term outcome. The process of cross-validation is expected to lead to reduction in the predictive power of a measuring instrument.

Three new raters were trained to use the Onset of Symptomatology Scale.* The raters were senior psychiatric residents who had no treatment or outcome information concerning the patient sample.

The hospital charts of the 120 patients contained in the Main Study were examined, and the following portions were reproduced for inclusion in a separate, de-identified Patient Research Folder:

1) The psychiatric intake review is a report dictated by the hospital admitting psychiatrist. It describes the patient and the parents at the time of admission and contains the stated reasons for admission, behavioral observations, a brief history, and mental status examination findings.

2) The social history is dictated by the social worker responsible for interviewing the patient's parents at the time of admission. It provides more detailed information about the nature of the referral, the patient's current living situation, childhood development, family background, dating information, educational, vocational, and avocational background, social relationships, and the social worker's observations, conclusions, and recommendations.

3) A complete psychological evaluation is conducted on each patient

---

*Fred L. Griffin, M.D., L. Dwight Holden, M.D., and David G. Oldham, M.D.

and contains psychodiagnostic and psychodynamic formulations, with accompanying treatment recommendations.

4) The initial evaluation staffing is conducted after admission. All past and present information is reviewed, diagnostic and dynamic formulations are constructed, and a treatment plan is formulated. These two-hour staff meetings are attended by the entire Adolescent Service team and are tape-recorded. The tape recordings are transcribed verbatim.

The Patient Research Folders specifically omit information about the patient's course in the hospital, the circumstances of the patient's discharge from the hospital, or any follow-up information subsequently obtained.

Table 14 presents interrater reliability correlations.

Subscale rater correlations range from .46 to .85, while the raters' correlations for the total score were .74, .75, and .77. These correlations are statistically significant. The psychiatric residents received approximately two hours of training in the use of the scale, and their level of reliability is roughly equivalent to that of the scale developer and an experienced child psychiatrist.

Subscale intercorrelations are presented in Table 15.

The subscales relate in a low to moderate fashion with each other,

TABLE 14

Interrater Reliability on the Onset of Symptomatology Scale*

| | Rater Pair | | |
Subscale	A–B	A–C	B–C
Psychological Trauma	.63	.70	.71
Physical Trauma	.79	.61	.59
Behavior Control	.51	.49	.57
Academic Progress	.76	.85	.75
Peer Relationships	.65	.78	.67
Passivity-Aggressiveness Deviance	.46	.49	.53
Symptom Duration	.68	.57	.54
Total Score	.75	.77	.74

*Pearson Product Moment Correlation Coefficients; $p < .01$
$N = 120$

TABLE 15

Subscale Intercorrelations for the Onset of Symptomatology Scale*

Subscale	(1)	(2)	(3)	(4)	(5)	(6)	(7)	(8)
(1) Psychological Trauma		.01	.13	.09	.42	.20	.32	.53
(2) Physical Trauma			.28	.27	.09	.05	.14	.48
(3) Behavior Control				.18	.32	.22	.34	.61
(4) Academic Progress					.17	.08	.36	.58
(5) Peer Relationships						.10	.47	.63
(6) Passivity-Aggressiveness Deviance							.21	.45
(7) Symptom Duration								.70
(8) Total Scale Score								—

*Pearson Product Moment Correlation Coefficients
$N = 120$

which suggests they are tapping different dimensions. Each subscale seems to contribute meaningfully to the overall score.

The crucial consideration, however, is the scale's relationship to outcome. These data are presented in Table 16.

Only two of the subscales (Psychological Trauma and Symptom Duration) are related to outcome level of function at a statistically significant level. This finding emphasizes the importance of cross-validation of clinically derived scales.

As in the Pilot Study, the total scores are highly differentiating at the reactive end. Most (37 of 48) patients with reactive scores attained Adaptive level of function ratings at follow-up; however, of the 57 patients scoring in the process range of the scale, 35 are rated Adaptive at outcome and 22 Poor. Thus, the Onset of Symptomatology Scale has some utility for predicting Adaptive outcome among reactive patients, but loses its ability to discriminate among patients with more chronically disturbed life histories. In both its overall degree of relationship to long-term outcome and its tendency to discriminate better for healthier patients than for more disturbed ones, the Onset of Symptomatology Scale appears similar to process-reactive and social competence scales developed for adults.[4]

Finally, combining information obtained from the Pilot Study and the Main Study, it appears that the Onset of Symptomatology Scale might be improved by deleting the Physical Trauma, Behavior Control, and Passivity-Aggressiveness Deviance subscales. These subscales show a weak relationship to outcome in the Pilot Study and essentially no relationship to outcome in the Main Study. In addition, they are among the subscales with lowest interrater reliability.

TABLE 16

Contingency Tables of Onset of Symptomatology Subscales
on Level of Function at Follow-Up

			Outcome	
Subscale	Score	n	Adaptive	Poor
Psychological Trauma	≤ 2	58	44	14
	≥ 3	47	28	19
	$X^2 = 3.20, p < .05$			
Physical Trauma	≤ 0	53	37	16
	≥ 1	52	35	17
	$X^2 = .08, p = $ n.s.			
Behavior Control	≤ 1	55	38	17
	≥ 2	50	34	16
	$X^2 = .01, p = $ n.s.			
Academic Progress	≤ 1	66	48	18
	≥ 2	39	24	15
	$X^2 = 1.42, p = $ n.s.			
Peer Relationships	≤ 1	40	30	10
	≥ 2	65	42	23
	$X^2 = 1.24, p = $ n.s.			
Passivity-Aggressiveness Deviance	≤ 2	53	37	16
	≥ 3	52	35	17
	$X^2 = .08, p = $ n.s.			
Symptom Duration	≤ 2	64	49	15
	≥ 3	41	23	18
	$X^2 = 4.86, p < .025$			
Total Score	≤ 12	48	37	11
	≥ 13	57	35	22
	$X^2 = 2.97, p < .05$			

FAMILY LEVEL OF COMPETENCE

Both clinical experience and the review of the literature suggest that patients' families have a powerful impact upon treatment process and outcome. Although the Social History Reports provided to the treatment staff by the team social worker were rich in clinical usefulness, they do not lend themselves to quantification that will allow comparison of families. Accordingly, a structured, videotaped family interview involving a series of tasks for each family to perform was designed. In an initial evaluation of 12 adolescent patient families and 11 control families, raters blind to the patient or nonpatient status of the family attained excellent interrater reliability viewing the videotaped family interactions. Interrater reliability coefficients ranged from .65 to .90, varying directly with the amount of family videotape material viewed and the level of clinical experience of the judges. Low but positive correlations were obtained between family level of competence and an independently derived measure of the adolescent patient's severity of psychopathology. Also, evaluations of the parental couple based on a task that involved the couple only correlated significantly with independent evaluations of the entire family working together.[6] Following this initial study, methodological improvements in the family testing procedure resulted in a five-part 50-minute format for family videotaped evaluations:

1) *Family strengths.* The family is asked to discuss as a group, "What is strong about your family?" They are informed they have 10 minutes for this discussion. The directions for this task, as for all of the other family tasks, are presented by tape recorder. (In the prior study the presence of an interviewer tended to change or disrupt family interactions.)

2) *Threatened loss.* A brief audiotape-recorded vignette portraying a hospital scene in which an unidentified male family member appears to be in imminent danger of dying is presented to the family. The vignette stops on an ambiguous note. The family members then are asked to make up an ending to the story in a 10-minute discussion.

3) *Marital testing.* With the children in another room, the parents

are asked to discuss, "What has been the best and the worst in your marriage?"

4) *Family closeness.* In this task, which involves all family members, they are asked to "discuss what closeness means in your family."

5) *Plan something together.* The family members are asked to plan a family activity which should be something they might actually do, which would involve all members of the family and would take at least an hour to perform.

The resulting family interactional videotape contains 40 minutes of full family interaction and 10 minutes of discussion between the parental couple with the children absent. Raters were asked to use the Beavers-Timberlawn Family Evaluation Scale* which had been developed during and after the pilot study family evaluation work described above.

The Family Evaluation Scale contains 13 subscales designed to assess the following: the family's power structure; quality of the parental coalition; closeness among family members; the nature of the family's shared beliefs concerning themselves; their ability to engage in efficient negotiation and problem-solving; clarity of disclosure of feelings and thoughts; the degree to which the family members take responsibility for their actions; their tendency to speak for each other; the degree of receptivity to each other's statements; family affective expressiveness; the overall mood and tone of the family interaction; the degree of unresolvable conflict displayed; and their ability to respond empathically to one another.

Finally, the raters made a Global Health-Pathology assessment on a scale from 1 (healthiest) to 10 (most pathological). Subsequent evaluation of 70 families containing an adolescent patient and 33 control families selected for competent functioning confirmed the previous finding that independent raters agree to a statistically significant degree concerning the level of family functioning. Ratings of family level of functioning of the same 70 patient-containing families cor-

---

*Appendix C

relate .52 ($p < .005$) with independent ratings of the severity of psycho-pathology of the adolescent on the Adolescent Psychopathology Scale.

All of the above Family Evaluation Scale data have been reported previously.[1,5,6,12] The Family Evaluation Scale has been used in a variety of subsequent studies unrelated to the Adolescent Treatment Assessment Project. It is clear that this is not a simple scale to teach to clinically unsophisticated raters, but we continue to obtain interrater reliability coefficients ranging from .49 to .88 for adequately trained, clinically sophisticated raters.

The various family evaluation subscales typically show low to moderate correlations with each other, and all tend to contribute in a meaningful way to the Global Health-Pathology ratings.

Table 17 demonstrates the relationship of family evaluation scores to subsequent adolescent patient follow-up level of function.

The raters (in addition to the senior author) include a senior psychiatrist, a nurse, two sociologists, and a psychiatric social worker.* The number of families observed for each rater varies as they each conducted their ratings for different clinical or research purposes. Family evaluations using this scale were begun late in the accumulation of data on the Main Study sample. Changes in certain subscales during the process of scale development further reduced data available for analysis.

While the analysis of these early data do not yield statistically significant findings, the strong trend noted for raters A and F (in which healthier family scores at the time of the patient's admission to the hospital do discriminate in the right direction for those former patients who attain an Adaptive level of function at follow-up) suggests that with a larger sample and some additional refinement in the scales themselves, assessment of family level of function could prove to have prognostic significance.

Two issues need emphasis. The family ratings were made shortly af-

---

*F. David Barnhart, M.A., W. Robert Beavers, M.D., Margie W. Buell, M.S.S.W., A.C.S.W., Susan B. Lewis, M.A., and Barbara W. Neill, R.N., M.S.

TABLE 17

Contingency Tables of Family Evaluation Scores and Level of Function at Follow-up: Six Raters

	Sum of Subscales Outcome			Global Health Pathology Outcome		
Score	Adaptive	Poor		Score	Adaptive	Poor
			Rater A			
≤ 47.5	9	2		≤ 8	23	7
≥ 48.0	8	5		≥ 9	7	6
			Rater B			
≤ 40.5	14	4		≤ 7	15	6
≥ 41.0	10	8		≥ 8	9	6
			Rater C			
≤ 45.0	6	1		≤ 7	5	3
≥ 45.5	6	3		≥ 8	7	1
			Rater D			
≤ 50.5	5	1		≤ 8	6	2
≥ 51.0	4	3		≥ 9	3	2
			Rater E			
≤ 52.5	8	1		≤ 8	15	5
≥ 53.0	6	1		≥ 9	11	4
			Rater F			
≤ 47.0	5	1		≤ 8	16	4
≥ 47.5	4	2		≥ 9	5	4

Chi Square analyses not significant.

ter admission and do not, therefore, reflect changes in the family as a consequence of family therapy. To expect a significant correlation of pre-therapy *family* ratings with patient outcome five years later may well be an unrealistic test of the importance of family factors.

The second issue is that, with rare exception, all of the families are rated as significantly dysfunctional, and they occupy but a narrow range on the Global Health-Pathology continuum. To expect to find predictive significance in such modest differences in family ratings is also a severe test of the importance of family factors.

LOCUS OF CONTROL

The Internal-External Locus of Control Scale is a forced choice, 29-item scale designed to measure an individual's feelings of control over his or her fate.[9] The items deal with beliefs about the nature of the world; that is, they are concerned with expectations about how rewards or reinforcements occur. The subject reads a pair of statements and then indicates with which of the two he or she more strongly agrees. "Internally controlled" individuals evidence the consistent belief that rewards generally derive from their own behavior; that is, that they can influence their environment. "Externally controlled" people, on the other hand, feel that rewards or punishments come to them much more often as a result of luck or chance; that is, that they have little influence over their environment.

The history of the Locus of Control Scale, extensive reliability data, and a wide range of research validation have been published.[9]

Staff working with hospitalized adolescents often find themselves frustrated by the teenagers' tendencies to blame other persons, circumstances, or fate for difficulties which result from their own behavior. Psychodynamically, these tendencies are generally referred to as denial, minimization, rationalization, and projection of blame. The frequency of such behaviors, particularly among adolescent inpatients with personality disorders, suggests that a measure of internal versus external locus of control might have predictive power for this group.

The Locus of Control Scale was used only during the hospitalization of the final 60 patients. Data presented in Table 18 indicate that patients obtaining an "internal" score attain a much higher level of func-

TABLE 18

Internal-External Locus of Control and Level of Function at Follow-up

Locus of Control	Level of Function	
	Adaptive	Poor
Internal ≤ 10	24	6
External ≥ 11	17	13

$X^2 = 2.8, p < .05$

tion at follow-up. Among those at the "external" end of the scale, a familiar phenomenon emerges—approximately a 50-50 distribution of Adaptive versus Poor outcome.

The strong relationship observed between Locus of Control scores and Follow-up Level of Function suggests that this brief, easy-to-administer test is a valuable addition to a predictive battery.[2,8]

SUMMARY AND OVERVIEW

The clinical scale instruments developed to evaluate adolescent patients' severity of psychopathology and chronicity of symptomatology relate significantly to the patients' five-year posthospital level of function. Correlations with measures of level of family competence are not statistically significant, but warrant further work. In addition, the Locus of Control Scale is a powerful addition to the predictive battery.

The predictive power of the Adolescent Psychopathology Scale can be approximately duplicated through the use of a single subscale, Diagnostic Severity. The revised Onset of Symptomatology Scale (containing subscales of the assessment of Psychological Trauma, Academic Progress, Peer Relationships, and Symptom Duration) improves upon the original and longer version of that scale.

All four scales described in this chapter discriminate better at the "healthier" end; that is, Adaptive outcome is attained by the majority of former patients with less severe psychopathology, more recent onset, less dysfunctional families of origin, and an internal locus of control. Each scale, however, loses much of its predictive power when assessing patients with more profound psychopathology.

REFERENCES

1. Beavers, W. R. *Psychotherapy and Growth: A Family Systems Perspective.* New York: Brunner/Mazel, 1977.
2. Davis, D. M., Gonzales, V., & Piat, J. Follow-up of adolescent psychiatric inpatients. *Southern Medical Journal,* 1980, *73,* 1215–1220.
3. Endicott, J., Spitzer, R. L., Fleiss, J. L., & Cohen, J. The global assessment scale: A procedure for measuring overall severity of psychiatric disturbance. *Archives of General Psychiatry,* 1976, *33,* 766–771.
4. Kokes, R. F., Strauss, J. S., & Klorman, R. Premorbid adjustment in schizo-

phrenia. II. Measuring premorbid adjustment: The instruments and their development. *Schizophrenia Bulletin,* 1977, *3,* 186–213.

5. Lewis, J. M. *How's Your Family?* New York: Brunner/Mazel, 1979.
6. Lewis, J. M., Beavers, W. R., Gossett, J. T., & Phillips, V. A. *No Single Thread: Psychological Health in Family Systems.* New York: Brunner/Mazel, 1976.
7. Luborsky, L. Clinicians' judgments of mental health. A proposed scale. *Archives of General Psychiatry,* 1962, *7,* 407–417.
8. Nowicki, S., & Strickland, B. R. A locus of control scale for children. *Journal of Consulting and Clinical Psychology,* 1973, *40,* 148–154.
9. Phares, E. J. *Locus of Control in Personality.* Morristown, N.J.: General Learning Press, 1976.
10. Rogler, L. H., & Hollingshead, A. B. *Trapped: Families and Schizophrenia.* New York: John Wiley & Sons, 1965.
11. Sampson, H., Messinger, S. L., & Towne, R. D. *Schizophrenic Women: Studies in Marital Crises.* New York: Atherton Press, 1964.
12. Usdin, G., & Lewis, J. M. *Psychiatry in General Medical Practice.* New York: McGraw-Hill, 1979.

CHAPTER 7

Treatment Process Correlates of Outcome

The treatment process and its relationship to outcome is an area of maximum interest to practicing clinicians, but poses great difficulties for the researcher. The methodological problems involved in distinguishing the influence of specific parts of a complex, diversified treatment program are staggering. In addition, potential interference in treatment planning and in the process of treatment itself by research personnel may prevent many projects from being conducted.

Examination of the treatment process was not a major goal of this project. Such an examination would have required additional personnel and funding that were not available. The clinical process within individual psychotherapy is itself an extremely complex and as yet poorly understood phenomenon. For example, Greenspan and Sharfstein recently have proposed an innovative paradigm for process evaluation of psychotherapy involving careful assessment of specific therapy goals, patient symptoms and developmental level, treatment trial therapist-patient interactions, alliance relationship variables, and outcome.[4]

Broadening this perspective to include group and family therapy, school and activities, interactions with unit staff, and the additional components of milieu therapy is outside the scope of this investigation. Such an ambitious project remains a goal for the future. Having measured patient, family, and post-discharge correlates of outcome, however, we think it is important to approach some aspects of the hospital treatment experience itself. To deal with the complexities of the treatment process by focusing on but a few treatment variables represents an unavoidable simplification.

The issue of potential interference in the treatment process has been met in two ways. One is to focus upon measures that are unobtrusive; the other is to collect research data in such a way that their immediate clinical usefulness is so great that the research is seen as a valuable addition to the treatment program, despite the intrusion. One example of each approach will be examined in this chapter.

Recording patterns of medication and assessing the relationship between these patterns and other patient and treatment variables as they influence outcome is an approach that is unobtrusive because all medications are routinely recorded by unit nurses. This information may be retrieved by research staff without interfering with the treatment process. Also, since medications are impersonal in nature (relative to psychotherapy or other verbal or behavioral staff-patient interactions), their study is less likely to arouse staff resistance.

The area of interpersonal relationships is one in which research personnel may gather data that can provide both on-the-spot clinical usefulness and yet have the potential for correlation with other patient and treatment variables of interest to the researcher. Although most psychiatric hospital programs make the quality of interpersonal relationships a major treatment focus, this is especially true in long-term programs that aim to go beyond relieving symptoms to changing relationship skills. Data gathered on interpersonal relationships in the hospital will be explored following an examination of patterns of medication usage.

PATTERNS OF MEDICATION USAGE*

Only four of the adolescent follow-up studies reviewed in Chapter 2 report the relationship of medication patterns to outcome. In the re-

---

*Medication data for this study were collected and analyzed by Karen Cassidy, R.N.

port by Hartmann and colleagues,[5] neither the administration, the type (minor tranquilizer, major tranquilizer, or antidepressant), nor the duration of medication use related to five-year outcome. In a later 10-year follow-up of the same patient group, however, use of medications during hospitalization is strongly associated with Poor long-range outcome.[6]

A similar finding was obtained by Garber,[3] who notes,

The use of medications of any type during the hospital course was associated with low functioning on follow-up. There was no differentiation between the type of medications used; all types were included. The absence of medications in the hospital was associated with high functioning on follow-up (p. 142).

Finally, Aarkrog, et al.[1] report that those who received medications in their study had significantly poorer outcome than those who did not. Thus, three recent studies agree that *any* use of medications with adolescents in a long-term treatment program is associated with poorer prognosis, but that duration of medication (constant versus sporadic) and type of medication used have not been demonstrated to relate to outcome.

Data are reported here on a sample of 81 Timberlawn adolescent patients for whom scores on a variety of other scales are available. All chart medication data were examined, and each patient was categorized in the following medication patterns:

1) No administration of psychotropic medications during hospitalization
2) Use of medications for one or more short-term periods (continuous use four weeks or less):
   (a) Sedatives only
   (b) Minor tranquilizers only
   (c) Major tranquilizers only
   (d) Antidepressants only
   (e) Any combination of drugs from two or more of the above categories
3) Continuous administration of medications for more than four weeks at a time:

(a) Sedatives only
(b) Minor tranquilizers only
(c) Major tranquilizers only
(d) Antidepressants only
(e) Any combination of drugs from two or more of the above
    categories

In addition, among the 10 patterns of medication usage each patient was coded by medication dose level. Medication dose equivalencies and the differentiation between "low" and "high" levels of medication are derived from Davis[2] and from consultation with two psychiatrists not connected with the research project who have special expertise in psychopharmacology.*

This categorization of medication dose levels is admittedly arbitrary, yet useful to differentiate those receiving small amounts of medication from those receiving large doses of one or more medications.**

The number of patients in each medication category is presented in Table 19.

Following an examination of the predictive value of medication variables, the relationship of significant aspects of medication use to other patient, family, and treatment characteristics will be analyzed. Medical records describing medication patterns were selected for those cases in which a variety of other characteristics were available. As a result, this group only partially overlaps the follow-up sample. Follow-up was available for 48 patients.

Following the lead of the investigators who find that any type of medication forecasts poor prognosis,[1,3,6] these 48 patients are categorized along that variable as demonstrated in Table 20.

Although the results of this analysis are in the expected direction, the differences are not statistically significant. Analysis of medications by type also proved nonsignificant. Comparison of patients receiving lower dose levels of medication versus higher dose levels of medication shows statistically nonsignificant results. Theoretically, patients re-

---

*Gregory Dimijian, M.D., and Larry E. Tripp, M.D.
**The dose equivalencies and levels are tabulated in Appendix E.

TABLE 19

Number of Patients in Medication Categories

Medication Category	Number of Patients
1. No medications	22
2. Short-term medications	
a. Sedatives only—low dosage	4
—high dosage	4
b. Minor tranquilizer only—low dosage	1
c. Major tranquilizer only—low dosage	5
d. Combinations—low dosage	3
—high dosage	3
3. Long-term medications	
a. Minor tranquilizer—low dosage	1
b. Major tranquilizer—low dosage	3
c. Combinations—low dosage	28
—high dosage	7

$N = 81$

TABLE 20

Medication of Patients with Adaptive and Poor Level of Function at Follow-Up

		Level of Function	
	n	Adaptive	Poor
Type of Medication			
No medication	12	10	2
Medication	36	22	14
(Sedatives only	3	2	1)
(Minor tranquilizer	2	1	1)
(Major tranquilizer	4	3	1)
(Combination	27	16	11)
	$X^2 = 2.46, p = $ n.s.		
Dose Level			
No medication	12	10	2
Low	28	17	11
High	8	5	3
	$X^2 = 2.02, p = $ n.s.		
Duration			
No medication	12	10	2
Short-term	12	10	2
Long-term	24	12	12
	$X^2 = 6.0, p < .025$		

ceiving medications of two or more different types might be presumed
to be of poorer prognosis, but this does not prove to be the case.

Finally, the data may be categorized by those patients who received
medications for one or more periods of less than four weeks at a time,
versus those patients who received medications for continuous periods
of longer than four weeks.

These results suggest that in this treatment program patients receiving no medications or only short-term prescriptions attain significantly better outcome levels of functioning than do those patients who receive medications for longer periods of time. Most (12) of the 16 patients with Poor long-term level of functioning were in the continuous
medication category.

No prior adolescent follow-up studies relate medication patterns to
other patient, family, or treatment variables, except the very global
finding that the more severely disturbed patients are more likely to be
given medications. In the present sample, the relationship of duration
of medication to diagnostic categories demonstrates a significant correlation in the expected direction (Table 21).

All psychotic patients in the sample were on medications for long
periods of time; personality disorder and neurotic patients were distributed among the categories of no medication, short-term, and long-
term. Assessment of other correlates of duration of medication did not
lead to statistically significant findings. However, when the sample included all 81 patients for whom medication patterns are available,
several correlates of duration of medication usage emerge: More male
patients received long-term medication, and a greater proportion of
female patients received no medication or short-term prescriptions.
This finding, however, is to some degree an artifact of the beliefs of the
prescribing physicians involved, a point to be considered carefully in
any analysis of the relationship of medications to other clinical findings or to outcome.

Dr. B prescribed long-term medications for two-thirds of his male
patients, but Dr. C gave either no medications or very brief prescriptions to approximately two-thirds of his female patients. Dr. A, also
an administrative psychiatrist for male patients, prescribed in a pattern
approximately midway between the other physicians. Personal communications with each psychiatrist suggest that their patterns of medi-

TABLE 21

Correlates of Medication

Variable	n	None	Short-Term	Long-Term
		Duration of Medication		
Diagnosis				
Neurosis	9	1	1	7
Personality Disorder	34	11	11	12
Psychosis	5	0	0	5
$X^2 = 10.90, p < .0025$				
Gender				
Male	47	8	12	27
Female	34	14	8	12
$X^2 = 6.37, p < .025$				
Administering Psychiatrist				
A (All male patients)	16	4	5	7
B (All male patients)	31	4	7	20
C (All female patients)	34	14	8	12
$X^2 = 8.2, p < .05$				
Diagnosis				
Neurosis	9	1	1	7
Personality Disorder	63	21	18	24
Psychosis	9	0	1	8
$X^2 = 11.97, p < .0125$				
Adolescent Psychopathology Scale Scores				
≤ 133	29	12	7	10
134–143	23	3	7	13
≥ 144	23	5	3	15
$X^2 = 8.33, p < .05$				
Length of Hospitalization				
≤ 273 days	19	6	5	8
274–591 days	32	8	13	11
≥ 592 days	30	8	2	20
$X^2 = 11.0, p < .025$				

cation prescription are influenced by differing beliefs about the appropriate use of medication in general, rather than being related entirely to symptomatic behaviors of the patients involved.

Other correlates, all variations of severity of psychopathology, emerge in the larger sample.

As noted before with the sample of 48 patients, most (eight out of nine) psychotic patients receive long-term medications, while the majority (39 out of 63) of personality disorder patients either received no medications or short-term prescriptions. Among the small number of patients given a neurotic diagnosis, most experienced marked anxiety and/or depression for long periods of time, and thus were medicated for long periods of time.

The relationship of duration of medications to patients' scores on the Adolescent Psychopathology Scale shows that patients receiving lower (less disturbed) scores on the Adolescent Psychopathology Scale tend to receive no medications or short-term prescriptions. Slightly more than half of the patients in the midrange of severity receive long-term medications, while a larger majority of patients with scores reflecting more profound psychopathology are given medications for long periods of time.

Finally, the relationship between duration of medication and hospital length of stay reveals that of patients hospitalized for shorter periods of time, approximately half receive long-term medications, while two-thirds of the longer stay patients receive medications for extended periods of time.

Returning to the subsample of 48 patients for whom follow-up data are available to examine the symptoms and behavioral signs for which medications are prescribed clarifies the relationships between medication prescriptions, patient behavior, and long-term outcome. For example, among the 20 patients who receive either no medications or brief periods of medication, and who have Adaptive outcome, none are psychotic, only one has an antisocial personality disorder diagnosis, and over half of the group have a secondary diagnosis of depression. In addition, only three of the group of 20 are noted to have preexisting drug-dependency problems. In the majority of these patients, medications were prescribed for acute anxiety or sleep disturbance. Thus, this group receiving little or no medications and achieving

Adaptive outcome comprises predominantly patients with milder personality disorder diagnoses, secondary depression, no thinking disorder, and transient problems with anxiety or sleep disturbance.

A small group of four patients who also received little or no medication, but who attained Poor long-term outcome contains two youngsters with antisocial personality disorder diagnoses without depressive symptoms. Most (three out of four) were noted to be drug-dependent before hospitalization. Medications for these four patients were prescribed for the control of physically violent episodes. Thus, the group of patients with Poor long-term outcome and brief medication usage were primarily antisocial and drug-dependent youngsters who had brief episodes of overt aggression during hospitalization.

A group of 12 patients receiving long-term medications who nevertheless attained Adaptive eventual outcome contains only one psychotic youngster and none with an antisocial personality disorder diagnosis. Ten had a secondary diagnosis of depression, and only two had prior drug-dependency problems. By and large, this is a group of personality disorder patients with depression, the majority of whom also demonstrated transient signs of thinking disturbances. Medications were given to these patients for chronic anxiety, chronic depression, sleep disturbance, and intermittent problems with cognitive slippage.

Finally, a subgroup of 12 patients receiving medications for long periods of time who later demonstrated Poor long-term outcome contains four youngsters with a psychotic diagnosis. Only three had a secondary diagnosis of depression. This is primarily a profoundly disturbed group who were given medications for both physical violence and long-term thinking disorder. About one-third of this group were chronically psychotic, while the other two-thirds currently would be diagnosed as severe borderlines. The most outstanding characteristics of this group are frequent violent episodes and either prolonged thinking disorders or numerous brief psychotic episodes.

The relationships between medication patterns and long-term outcome appear to relate to different ideologies about the use of medications. If the predominant treatment philosophy is that medications are used only for chronic thinking disorder or behavioral control of violent aggressive episodes, then use of medications correlates with Poor outcome as they are given primarily to poor prognosis patients.

If the treatment philosophy, however, *also* involves the use of medications on a short-term basis for intermittent severe anxiety, phobic reactions, and acute depressive episodes, the use of medications does not correlate with outcome. In such cases, duration of medication usage becomes the critical variable in the prediction of outcome.

The importance of ideology is highlighted in the setting in which these data were obtained. Although the basic ideology is psychoanalytic, unit psychiatrists differ in their thinking about the role of psychotropic medications in the total treatment process. As a consequence, there are, as illustrated in Table 21, significant differences in the ways in which medications are prescribed, and these differences confound the relationship between use of medication and the outcome of treatment.

INTERPERSONAL RELATIONSHIPS*

A major focus of many inpatient treatment programs (and certainly of any intermediate to long-term program) is the nature and quality of patients' interpersonal relationships. Much of the verbal interaction taking place between staff and patients centers around issues such as friendship choices and styles of relating to peers and to staff. Often very focused examination of interpersonal behaviors that enhance or interfere with the establishment and maintenance of close, meaningful, growth-promoting relationships occurs. In this context, it is striking that only one previous follow-up investigator reports data bearing on this issue.[3] In his examination of inpatient factors predictive of long-term outcome, Garber notes that a variable labeled "Involvement with the Adolescent Group" correlates significantly with former patients' posthospitalization level of function. It is unclear, however, whether this variable is based upon patients' ratings or upon staff's perception of the patients' involvement with their hospitalized peers.

This is an important distinction, because it has been demonstrated that peers' ratings of interpersonal involvement are better predictors of adult level of function than are teachers' or mental health professionals' ratings of child and adolescent peer involvement.[7] Among a group of youngsters evaluated as being at risk for later severe dysfunction,

---

*Data in this section were analyzed by William S. Logan, M.D.[8]

psychiatric predictions do not correlate with the later development of psychosis, but peers' ratings of interpersonal relationships do correlate with subsequent psychotic disorders.[7]

In addition, it seems that when adults (teachers or mental health professionals) evaluate children's or adolescents' peer relations they are heavily influenced positively by the appearance of sociability and poise and negatively by shyness or passivity. However, when children and adolescents rate each other on closeness of relationships, they are relatively uninfluenced by such factors and appear to form and maintain friendship patterns more on the basis of character traits such as moral maturity or responsibility, factors which subsequently prove to have much greater long-term predictive power.[7]

Reviewing a number of studies of heterogeneous groups of children and adolescents, Kohlberg et al.[7] state that intelligence and antisocial behavior are the strongest predictors of adult adjustment, with peer relationships running a close third. Peer acceptance during childhood and adolescence is a strong predictor of healthy adult adjustment, although peer rejection does not necessarily predict adult dysfunction.

At approximately three-month intervals between 1972 and 1974, all adolescent patients in the Timberlawn program listed the three fellow patients and the three staff members to whom they felt closest. At the time of each patient's "closeness" ratings, staff members also rank ordered the patients with whom they worked along a "closeness" dimension, from the patient to whom they felt closest to the patient from whom they felt most distant.

Immediately following each data collection, research staff organized the ratings and provided a five-to-10-page clinical summary of the findings to treatment team leaders. The following is a de-identified portion of one such "Closeness Report":

Summary of Girls' Data

Mutual Relationships

Four girls had all their peer choices reciprocated. These were *Jane, Betty, Sue,* and *Mary. Lisa* and *Shelly* had two choices reciprocated. *Tina, Jerri, Beth,* and *Debbie* had none of their choices reciprocated. On the last survey, *Tina* enjoyed three mutual choices. The number of mutual choices overall has remained constant over the last three surveys.

Popularity with Peers

Mary and *Betty* were each chosen by eight peers. *Sue* and *Jane* were chosen six and five times respectively. *Jerri* and *Beth* were not chosen. *Tina* dropped in popularity, having been chosen by five peers on the previous survey, and only one for this report.

Total Degree of Closeness to Staff

Four girls indicated they felt very close to the staff. *Mary* and *Jane* indicated they felt closer to three staff members than they have ever felt to anyone. *Tina* and *Beth* indicated great closeness to staff, in contrast to their peer distance. *Betty, Sue,* and *Debbie* showed the greatest distance from staff.

Selected Individual Summaries

Tina: Tina appears to fluctuate from one report to the next. From her admission until February, she showed gradual increases in closeness on all categories. By February, she was one of the most popular girls and showed three mutual relationships. Apart from her perceived closeness to staff, this report appears more like her earlier reports.

Jerri: This is Jerri's first report. She shows distance from peers and average closeness to staff. She was not chosen by her peers.

Laura: Laura has moved into the peer and staff groups for the first time since her admission. She shows average closeness to both, and was chosen by one of the more popular girls.

Betty: Betty has emerged on this report as a closeness "star," having great popularity. Her three choices were reciprocated. She, however, indicates distance from both peers and staff in her assessment of how close these friendships are.

Girls' Sociogram

The girls' group is more homogeneous than the last survey, with the one major group consisting of *Betty, Mary, Jane, Sue,* and *Lisa. Shelly* and *Laura* have peripheral membership in this group, with *Carol*

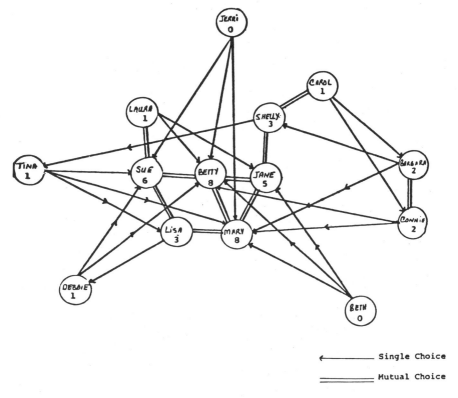

Figure 2. Adolescent Girls' Sociogram

ambivalent in choosing the dominant group or affiliating with the minor group of *Barbara* and *Connie*. *Jerri, Beth, Tina,* and *Debbie* are isolated from either group, but for the most part show one-way choices with girls from the dominant group.

Summary of Boys' Data

Mutual Relationships

Mutual relationships continue to decrease in number (there were 24 two surveys ago, 14 last survey, and 10 for this report). *Bob* had three mutual choices; *Al, John,* and *David* had two mutual choices. *Mike* had one choice reciprocated. The other seven boys showed no mutual choices.

Popularity with Peers

Bob and *Al* were chosen by nine and eight peers respectively. *Bill,* who was chosen 10 times on the last report, was not chosen by anyone for this survey. *David* was chosen by five peers. Four boys (*John, Mike, Tommy,* and *Jack*) were each chosen by three boys. *Jerry* and *Carl* were each chosen once, with the remaining three boys not being chosen.

Total Degree of Closeness to Staff

Tommy and *Al* display the greatest degree of closeness to staff, with *Bob, John, David,* and *Jack* showing slightly more than average degrees of closeness to staff. *Bill* and *Jerry* indicated the greatest distance from staff. *Jerry* has shown average degrees of closeness to staff in his past surveys.

Selected Individual Summaries

Bill: Bill demonstrates a most dramatic fall from leadership since the last report. In the previous report, Bill was chosen by all but one of his peers and was close to both peers and staff.

Mike: Mike shows increased closeness to peers since the last report. He enjoyed one mutual choice and was chosen by two popular boys.

Jerry: Jerry's distance from staff and patients has increased. He was chosen by only one peer.

Steve: Steve remains isolated over the past two surveys.

Al: Al has become quite popular among the adolescent boys, having been chosen by eight peers. He indicates that he is close to staff and has average closeness to peers.

Boys' Sociogram

The boys' sociogram shows a strong coalition in the center of *Al, Bob,* and *John,* with *David* and *Mike* on the periphery. The isolates remain much the same since the last report, although they show less tendency to choose the closeness leadership core, choosing *Jack, Tommy,* and *David. Bill* has lost his central position regarding closeness.

The content of these ratings and reports was further amplified in

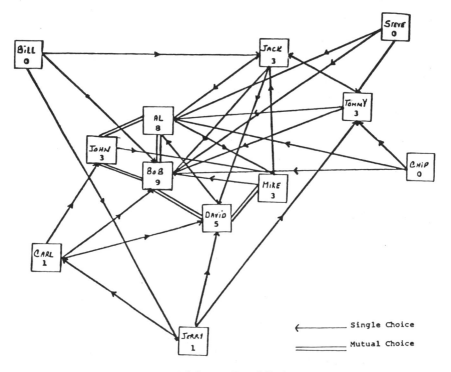

Figure 3. Adolescent Boys' Sociogram

staff discussions and frequently formed the basis for additional treatment interventions designed to improve relationship skills of youngsters noted to be deficient or to encourage and maintain the accomplishments of patients who appeared to be faring well in interpersonal relationships.

In some cases the research data appeared merely to confirm informal staff observations of relationships, but it was not uncommon for patterns of peer popularity, rejection, or subgrouping to emerge that were surprising and enlightening to treatment staff.

Clinically, ratings on any single closeness survey were useful; however, dramatic shifts in peer popularity, subgroup patterns, and number of close friendships occurred from one survey to another. These were due, in part, to extraneous factors such as discharges, new admissions, and the ebb and flow of group process on the treatment units.

For research purposes, data analysis is restricted to the 32 patients who
were involved in at least three consecutive surveys.

A primary measure of interpersonal relationships tapped by the
closeness surveys was *mutual relationships,* that is, any two adolescents independently choosing each other as one of their closest peer
friends. Table 22 shows the correlations between average number of
mutual relationships per survey and subsequent posthospital outcome
ratings.

The majority of youngsters who form and maintain reciprocated relationships experience Adaptive global outcome, while those who do
not form and maintain reciprocal relationships divide evenly on the
outcome measures. This finding essentially agrees with prior research.
In addition, mutual choices are significantly and positively related to
later independent assessments of Peer and Social Functioning at follow-up.

Popularity—that is, the number of times patients are chosen by their
peers—also predicts outcome as measured by peer relationships. This
repeats the pattern seen in regard to other variables in which the majority of popular youngsters achieve Adaptive long-term outcome. Those
who are not popular with peers during hospitalization are about equally divided between Adaptive and Poor outcome.

Turning to adolescent patients' perceptions of *closeness to staff,*
their ratings of feelings of closeness toward unit nurses predicts Adaptive outcome, but their feelings of closeness toward other staff members do not relate to long-term outcome.

At the time patients were evaluating their relationships to each other
and to staff, staff were ranking patients in the order of their own *feelings of closeness toward the patients.* It was striking that staff feelings
of closeness to the patients do *not* predict long-term outcome.

The meaningfulness of these interpersonal relationship ratings as
predictive variables is striking. Clearly data collected in this manner
have both immediate clinical usefulness in the planning and conduct of
a milieu treatment program and also powerful long-term predictive
significance.

These findings are of particular significance in view of the assumption of many treatment personnel that their affective reactions to patients contain greater prognostic power than patients' feelings toward

TABLE 22

Closeness Ratings and Outcome Level of Function

	Level of Function at Follow-up	
Closeness Selections	Adaptive	Poor

Follow-up Assessment of Global Functioning

Average number of mutual choices

>1	18	5
≤1	4	5

$X^2 = 2.05, p = $ n.s.

Popularity with peers

>Chosen 2.5 times	14	3
≤Chosen 2.5 times	8	7

$X^2 = 1.92, p = $ n.s.

Continuity of choice of staff

Chose same nurse at least 2 times	13	1
No consistent choice	9	9

$X^2 = 4.89, p < .025$

Staff perception of closeness to patients

Above median	11	5
Below median	11	5

$X^2 = .15, p = $ n.s.

Follow-up Assessment of Peer and Social Functioning

Average number of mutual choices

>1	18	5
≤1	3	6

$X^2 = 3.97, p < .025$

Popularity with peers

>Chosen 2.5 times	15	2
≤Chosen 2.5 times	6	9

$X^2 = 6.22, p < .0125$

$N = 32$

each other. Our findings with hospitalized adolescents appear to support data derived from the body of longitudinal studies exploring childhood predictors of adult mental health status. Kohlberg et al. state,

> In a certain sense, this evidence suggests that children are better diagnosticians than are adult clinicians, i.e., that their spontaneous evaluations of each other are more predictive than are the ratings of adults on mental health behavior (p. 1256).[7]

No definitive explanation is available for the superior long-term predictive value of adolescent peer relationship assessments over those made by adult clinicians. However, a partial explanation may derive from the observation that all such studies have been conducted in some form of institutional setting (hospital, school, or other residential or educational program). Within such settings, staff members' affective responses to a patient or student may be influenced by the youngster's apparent conformity to institutionalized goals and procedures. Adolescent peers' sociometric ratings of each other, however, may be sensitive to a broader range of more enduring and more meaningful personality characteristics.

Of related interest is the finding that adolescent patients' feelings of closeness toward unit nurses are predictive of later adult functioning, while their feelings toward other staff members do not predict outcome. This occurs in the context of a program strongly emphasizing the importance of the youngsters' relationships to their administrative psychiatrist, their psychotherapists, teachers, and other members of the treatment team. Within a highly organized, long-term milieu program, it may be the unit nurses who most clearly and positively reflect a combination of nurturance and control to which patients must respond. It is not surprising that an adolescent's ability to integrate these very different aspects of relationships with adults in a consistent, close relationship has important prognostic significance.

REFERENCES

1. Aarkrog, T., Lauritsen, S., Mortensen, K., & Strom, J. Adolescents in psychiatric residential treatment and five years later. *Acta Psychiatrica Scandinavica,* 1979, Supplement 278, Copenhagen.

2. Davis, J. M. Comparative doses and costs of antipsychotic medication. *Archives of General Psychiatry,* 1976, *33,* 858–861.
3. Garber, B. *Follow-up Study of Hospitalized Adolescents.* New York: Brunner/ Mazel, 1972.
4. Greenspan, S. A., & Sharfstein, S. S. Efficacy of psychotherapy: Asking the right questions. *Archives of General Psychiatry,* 1981, *38,* 1213–1219.
5. Hartmann, E., Glasser, B., Greenblatt, M., Solomon, M., & Levinson, D. *Adolescents in a Mental Hospital.* New York: Grune & Stratton, 1968.
6. Herrera, E. G., Lifson, B. G., Hartmann, E., & Solomon, M. H. A 10-year follow-up of 55 hospitalized adolescents. *American Journal of Psychiatry,* 1974, *131,* 769–774.
7. Kohlberg, L., LaCrosse, J., & Ricks, D. The predictability of adult mental health from childhood behavior. In B. B. Wolman (Ed.), *Manual of Child Psychopathology.* New York: McGraw-Hill, 1972, pp. 1217–1284.
8. Logan, W. S., Barnhart, F. D., & Gossett, J. T. The prognostic significance of adolescent interpersonal relationships during psychiatric hospitalization. In S. Feinstein, J. Looney, A. Schwartzberg, & A. Sorosky (Eds.), *Adolescent Psychiatry: Developmental and Clinical Studies,* (Vol. 10). Chicago: The University of Chicago Press, in press, 1982.

CHAPTER 8

Multivariate Predictions of Outcome

In this study, as in all previous ones except that reported by Garber,[1] the search for correlates of treatment outcome involves the process of relating a series of patient, family, and treatment variables to outcome level of function one at a time. This approach does identify discriminating variables, but it does not reflect fully the reality of clinical practice in which the variables interact with bewildering complexity.

It seems appropriate, therefore, to seek more complex multivariate assessments of treatment outcome. Before proceeding, however, several cautionary notes are in order. The size of the sample takes on greatly increased importance when attempting to combine predictor variables. Ideally, one has a very large sample of patients, all of whom have been evaluated by the same individual, family, and treatment measures. Under these conditions, multivariate statistical techniques might be expected to select from the mass of data those variables relating most meaningfully to eventual outcome. Realistic considerations, however, work against this optimal arrangement. Indepth outcome assessment requires individual examination of each subject (and a close family member) by a skilled clinician. Locating and assessing them in this manner is time-consuming and, therefore, very costly. As a result, most follow-up populations have contained rather small numbers. In addition, the "state of the art" in selection of variables to be measured and in the selection of specific scales for measuring these variables is such that awareness of the most promising variables and measures is likely to change during the course of a longitudinal study. New variables and improved measures become available after data collection has begun, and often it is not possible to apply new measurement techniques to "old" cases in a truly comparable manner.

After the Pilot Study, a commitment was made to obtain outcome assessment on at least 100 consecutive admissions, and that goal was accomplished. However, an additional commitment was made to a flexible, open approach to the measurement of patient, family, and treatment variables. That is, we knew that years would elapse between initial measurements and eventual outcome assessment, and we decided to adopt new predictor measures as they became available and to delete other variables when it became obvious that their usefulness was limited. This approach keeps one up-to-date with advances in clinical assessment, but it also results in substantial data loss, because later cases are assessed on some different dimensions than patients who move through the treatment program at earlier dates.

Multivariate statistical techniques may be applied to relatively small samples, but the confidence placed in the results decreases proportionately. As a consequence, we limit multivariate assessment to those predictor variables on which the sample size is at least 50. Even with this restriction, however, the results must be considered tentative. In our judgment, a sample size of at least 100 patients evaluated with the same individual, patient, and treatment measures provides a more acceptable base for making clear, confident statements concerning the relative importance of the predictor variables and their interactions. With this caveat, the data are presented, in part, to encourage others to improve on the present approach with a wider range of variables and larger patient samples.

The multivariate statistical technique probably best known to clinicians is stepwise multiple regression analysis (see Chapter 3) that examines the relationship of several predictor variables to an outcome measure simultaneously. It selects the best predictor, then adds additional predictors ranked in terms of the degree to which each contributes predictive power over and above those previously identified.

Stepwise discriminate analysis, a related statistical technique, ac-

complishes a similar task. However, it expresses the results in a way
that maximizes the difference on the dependent variable between two
or more groups of cases. Given the two groups of outcome (Adaptive
versus Poor), discriminate analysis identifies the combination of
weighted independent variables which best predicts a subject's group
membership. This technique seems well suited to the clinician's interest in accurate prediction early in treatment of those patients most likely to attain an Adaptive treatment outcome in contrast to those more
likely to have Poor long-term results. Increasing the clinician's ability
to make valid long-term outcome predictions is of obvious importance
in crucial decisions concerning whether or not to hospitalize a patient,
how best to organize an individual's treatment program, and how to
estimate necessary duration of treatment. The ability to provide empirically based information to patients, families, and funding sources
concerning the treatment interventions recommended can be strength-
ened.

INITIAL ASSESSMENT ANALYSIS

The best predictor variables available during the initial assessment
phase of treatment in this study were diagnostic level and scores on
scales measuring adolescent psychopathology, onset of symptomatology, family evaluation, and locus of control.

Although it is theoretically possible to convert DSM-II diagnoses into DSM-III equivalents, the major structural change from the single
axis DSM-II approach to the multiaxial DSM-III approach renders
these conversions suspect. Of the remaining measures, the Family
Evaluation Scale was the last to be developed and, although it is a promising clinical technique with obvious treatment planning implications,
the data reflect too small a sample to be included in a multivariate analysis. Accordingly, discriminate analysis was conducted with data on 59
patients with scores on the Onset of Symptomatology Scale, the Adolescent Psychopathology Scale, and the Locus of Control Scale. Tables 23 and 24 provide the results of the discriminate analysis using
these predictors. The a priori probability of classification in each
group is based on each group's size.

The results of this analysis suggest that the combination of Adoles-

TABLE 23

Variables Included in the Discriminant Function

| Predictor Variables | Discriminant Function Coefficient | | |
	Wilk's Lambda	Unstandardized Coefficient	Standardized Coefficient
1. Adolescent Psychopathology	.88	.054	.89
2. Locus of Control	.84	.124	.53
3. Onset of Symptomatology	—	—	—

Note. Constant Coefficient = − 8.59
$X^2 = 9.73, p < .008$

cent Psychopathology Scale and Locus of Control Scale scores maximizes the discrimination between Adaptive outcome and Poor outcome; Onset of Symptomatology scores add little to the predictive power of the two previous measures used in combination. Figure 4 illustrates the results.

The discriminate analysis correctly classified 76 percent of the sample into Global outcome categories. Referring to Figure 4, it may be seen that all patients with lower (less severe) scores on the Adolescent Psychopathology Scale and internal Locus of Control attained Adaptive outcome. Most patients (nine of 12) with less severe Adolescent Psychopathology scores and external Locus of Control also were found to be doing well at follow-up.

TABLE 24

Comparison of Classification Based on Global Outcome with Classification Based on the Discriminant Function Analysis (DFA) (Adolescent Psychopathology, Locus of Control)

| Global Outcome | DFA | | | |
| | Adaptive | | Poor | |
	N	(%)	N	(%)
Adaptive	38	(93)	3	(7)
Poor	11	(61)	7	(39)

Grouped Cases Correctly Classified = 76%

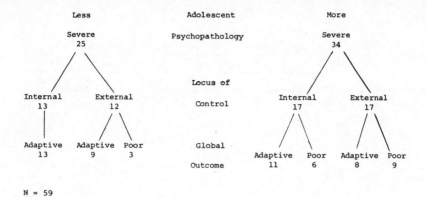

Figure 4. Global Outcome by Adolescent Psychopathology and Locus of Control

Among patients with more severe Adolescent Psychopathology Scale scores, 11 of 17 with internal Locus of Control have successful outcome, while those with external Locus of Control divide evenly on the outcome measure.

HOSPITAL DISCHARGE ANALYSIS

Among variables assessed during the course of treatment, completion of the recommended treatment program satisfies the criterion of at least 50 cases in which there is overlapping with other variables. Tables 25 and 26 contain the discriminate analysis relevant to the clinical issue of outcome prediction at the time of hospital discharge.

This discriminate analysis selects three predictor variables—scores on the Adolescent Psychopathology Scale, Locus of Control Scale, and the clinical judgment of Treatment Completion. The accuracy of prediction is not helped, however, by the addition of the completion of treatment measure. Figure 5 displays these results in visual form.

Although completion of treatment by itself is the best variable tested at the time of discharge, it does not add to predictive power when used in combination with the admission variables. In part this may be due to the very small number of cases in each outcome category when the total sample size is small and three predictor variables are used for

TABLE 25

Variables Included in the Discriminant Function

Predictor Variables	Wilk's Lambda	Unstandardized Coefficient	Standardized Coefficient
1. Completion of Treatment	.87	1.180	.56
2. Adolescent Psychopathology	.83	−.033	−.54
3. Locus of Control	.80	−.103	−.44
4. Onset of Symptomatology	—	—	—

Note. Constant Coefficient = 4.94
$X^2 = 12.57, p < .006$

classification. For example, when one examines patients with less severe Adolescent Psychopathology scores and external Locus of Control, only three patients fall in the subgroup failing to complete the recommended treatment program. The finding that two of these three have Poor long-term outcome carries little weight in contrast to what might be determined with a much larger subgroup.

For patients with more severe Adolescent Psychopathology scores and external Locus of Control, completion of treatment yields three of four successful outcomes, while failure to complete treatment results in eight of 13 Poor outcomes, but these numbers also are too small to be very meaningful for clinical prediction.

TABLE 26

Comparison of Classification Based on Global Outcome with Classification Based on the Discriminant Function Analysis (DFA) (Adolescent Psychopathology, Locus of Control, Completion of Treatment)

Global Outcome	DFA			
	Adaptive		Poor	
	N	(%)	N	(%)
Adaptive	36	(88)	5	(12)
Poor	10	(56)	8	(44)

Grouped Cases Correctly Classified = 75%

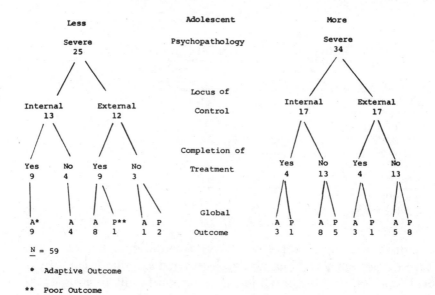

Figure 5. Global Outcome by Adolescent Psychopathology, Locus of Control, and Completion of Treatment

FOLLOW-UP ASSESSMENT ANALYSIS

Among the variables assessed during the post-discharge period, continuation of recommended psychotherapy in contrast to premature termination satisfies the criterion of 50 cases for whom all previous variables have also been assessed. However, the addition of continuation of psychotherapy does not improve the discriminate function analysis.

OVERVIEW OF MULTIVARIATE ANALYSES

The results of these analyses should not be interpreted to imply that other measures are clinically irrelevant. For example, analyses of single variables reported in Chapters 5, 6, and 7 strongly support the clinical usefulness of refined measures of Diagnostic Severity, Onset of Symptomatology, medication patterns, interpersonal relationships during hospitalization, and the continuation of psychotherapeutic treatment following discharge. Most of these variables are excluded from the multivariate analysis despite considerable promise, because of small sample size. The measures of chronicity of dysfunction and continuation of psychotherapy following discharge are excluded statistically from the analyses because they add little to the predictive power of combinations of other measures. This may indicate that they are, in fact, weak prognostic variables, yet another equally plausible interpretation is that the variables themselves simply correlate with other powerful variables in this sample. It is also possible that the clinical scales developed to measure these variables require additional refinement to increase their predictive power.

Such issues can be resolved empirically through the application of refined scaling techniques to larger patient samples. Given the vagaries of human behavior and our present limited powers of reliable assessment, the clinician's ability early in the treatment course to make prognostic statements reaching five to 10 years into the future (at a 76 percent degree of accuracy) with the rather crude clinical measures currently available is no small accomplishment.

While it is likely that other patterns of predictor variables will offer more accurate prognostic statements in different treatment settings, empirical knowledge of these maximum prognostic patterns awaits replication in such settings. Informal exchange with research clinicians in other settings offers the hope that within the next decade hospital mental health professionals not only will be able to make much more accurate prognostic statements, but also will have accumulated a considerable body of data bearing on the most meaningful clinical issue of improved matching of treatment approaches to patient and family needs.

REFERENCE

1. Garber, B. *Follow-up Study of Hospitalized Adolescents.* New York: Brunner/Mazel, 1972.

PART III

Clinical and Research Implications

CHAPTER 9

Clinical Implications
for Improved
Hospital Treatment

Ultimate justification for conducting follow-up treatment assessment research lies in three areas: 1) increased knowledge of treatment effects and, therefore, treatment planning and prognosis provided to practicing clinicians; 2) positive impact on staff morale; and 3) the usefulness of information in accountability. This chapter focuses primarily on the first of these, although a few comments are in order about the others.

Many of these findings have been presented to clinicians in a variety of hospital settings. The impression has been that this information has had a positive impact on staff morale—energizing, sustaining, and directing them in their day-to-day work. While accountability purposes are often served more directly by traditional hospital practices such as Utilization Review, Medical Audit, Quality Assurance, and constant emphasis on the importance of documentation, the type of information contained in this chapter supports and informs hospital staff and, in that sense, contributes to accountability.

To provide a context, it is important to indicate how the items in this chapter were selected. First, some of the data are derived directly from specific research methodologies and statistical demonstrations, but they are not limited to those findings. "Softer" sources of outcome information are included as well, because they have clinical significance.

Second, findings applicable to a variety of treatment programs—
short-term and long-term—existing in a variety of treatment institutions are presented. Despite variations, it is our impression that effective programs are basically more alike than different, and this summary of a variety of experiences gleaned from long-term follow-up
with former adolescent patients appears to be applicable to many inpatient settings.

Third, this description of findings is limited to those items explored
at follow-up assessment rather than including issues of treatment phi-
losphy which, although relevant to inpatient treatment planning, have
not been verified.

Finally, the items presented in this chapter are a representative, not
exhaustive, list. They supplement findings presented in Chapters 2
through 8. They are organized as items relating primarily to individual
patient care, items relating to families of inpatients, and findings with
staff or program implications.

INDIVIDUAL PATIENT FINDINGS

Varieties of Adaptive Outcome

It has long been known that patients with less severe psychopathology show higher treatment success rates than those with more
severe psychopathology, but greater prognostic specificity is possible.
The use of clinical scales of discrete processes sharpens prediction considerably over global assessments. Also, the long-term value of completing reasonable inpatient treatment goals and of continuing psychotherapeutic contacts following hospital discharge is emphasized. It is
especially striking that many youngsters who present with severe psychotic or personality disorder symptomatology can be effectively treated with lasting impact.

Case-by-case analysis indicates that the majority of youngsters with
less severe forms of psychopathology or with more recent onset do well
in a longer term program despite the failure of earlier treatment. For
example, combining the Pilot Study and Main Study groups, we note
that 18 of 20 patients who are given neurotic diagnosis obtain Adaptive
outcome regardless of their position on other variables. In addition,

dividing this 176-patient group into those with more recent onset versus those with more chronic onset (based upon their scores on the Onset of Symptomatology Scale), 45 of the 63 personality disorder and psychotic patients (71 percent) with more recent onset do well. In fact, almost all recent onset personality disorder and psychotic patients do well if they complete their inpatient treatment programs and continue psychotherapy after discharge.

Moving to those youngsters with more chronic psychopathology, the success rate is still striking; that is, about two-thirds of the chronic personality disorder patients demonstrated Adaptive outcome. Chronic psychotic patients, however, do not fare so well—only nine of 32 rate Adaptive at follow-up.

If we focus upon the two groups with most serious disturbances—the chronic psychotic and chronic personality disorders—several subgroups of such patients can be identified for whom clinicians might have predicted Poor outcome, but many of whom are rated at an Adaptive level. The largest subgroup is the long-term personality disorder adolescents with substantial amounts of antisocial behavior who demonstrate (often from the beginning of treatment): 1) subtle signs of genuine guilt and remorse concerning their behavior; 2) above average academic ability; and 3) realistic vocational aspirations.

Another subgroup are those functioning Adaptively through increased accommodation to the efforts of others. For example, several are maintained by spouses despite obvious ongoing psychopathology; and several are supported by an extensive family network which expects or demands little of the patient.

A still smaller subgroup contains those patients with severe continuing psychopathology who do better as young adults than as adolescents because of increased impulse control and modification of their pathology into vocational success. Several markedly schizoid persons, for example, maintain themselves by virtue of compulsive vocational skills and a comfortable degree of interpersonal isolation. Such individuals are able to support themselves economically, maintain sufficient superficial vocational and social relationships, and coexist fairly comfortably at some distance from their parents. In addition, there are several sociopathic youngsters who also succeed in life through increased impulse control and modulation of their personality characteristics into forms that allow vocational success. One such individual sells encyclopedias; one is a radio disc jockey; and another is an industrial manufacturer's representative. These former patients are alike in their high-powered sales abilities, and they work in fields where geographical mobility is not a disadvantage. They demonstrate little or no need for enduring interpersonal relationships and are able to stay out of serious trouble with alcohol, drugs, and the law. Thus, even among profoundly disturbed patients, one sees successful outcomes accomplished through mechanisms other than structural personality change.

Varieties of Poor Outcome

There also are identifiable subgroups of patients obtaining Poor long-term levels of function. The largest group still functioning poorly at five-year follow-up are the chronic personality disorder patients with antisocial features. Most of this group carry an antisocial diagnosis. Most are male and come from several familiar family constellations: 1) the chaotic, impulse-ridden family in which alcohol and/or drug abuse, running away, physical fights, and illegal acts are part of family life for several or all family members; 2) the "pillar-of-the community," rigid, puritanical, repressed family in which the patient is chronically rejected and severely scapegoated; or 3) the extremely rigid, conflict-habituated family.

Patients in this antisocial subgroup demonstrate lifelong histories of conflict with authority, peer relationships limited to similar others, marked academic underachievement, early delinquency, heavy reliance on alcohol and illicit drugs, and a continuation of an antisocial lifestyle into adulthood. While in the hospital, such youngsters continue to act out their authority conflicts with daily power struggles and rule breaking; often they run away from the hospital, sign out prematurely, or manipulate their parents into withdrawing them from the treatment program.

The second subgroup of Poor outcome patients are the chronic, severely schizophrenic adolescents who do not improve in adulthood. There are about equal numbers of males and females; they tend to remain in the treatment program much longer than the average—some for two-and-a-half to four years, as opposed to an average of about one year for the total population. Rehospitalizations or even continuous hospitalizations are common. These individuals demonstrated clear psychotic symptomatology at least since puberty. They are seen as different from youngsters with more reactive psychoses in that periods of nonpsychotic functioning tend to be rare and brief. They resist the effects of medication, support from hospital structure, and psychotherapy. They impress staff and peers alike as being highly stressed by the day-to-day demands of the treatment program, and are rarely, if ever, comfortable except when restricted to their rooms or physically restrained.

A final subgroup (predominantly girls) would be diagnosed currently as severe to profound borderlines. Their most striking shared characteristic is repetitive physical violence directed toward self or others. Some in this group have never been psychotic, while others show occasional brief psychotic episodes. All, however, demonstrate episodes of sudden physical violence when frustrated, deprived, or angered. Self-destructive acts committed by members of this group usually are described by the patient as "suicidal," but clinicians note a striking absence of overt depression and the clear presence of strong motives for revenge. Such vengeful acts seem directed toward parents (for placing the patient in the hospital or refusing to withdraw the patient from the hospital), toward staff (when frustrated by a restriction or by the absence of a desired staff person), or toward a peer (when envious of a visit, possession, or relationship). Physical attacks directed toward others occur most often in the context of disputes in which staff members are attempting to make the patient go to school or accept a restriction.

Following discharge, such youngsters often attain periods of several weeks or months of tenuous adaptation, but new episodes of physical violence, psychotic periods, rehospitalizations, and other severe medical, legal, and interpersonal disturbances are common. When followed over a 10-15-year span, there are striking outcome similarities between these "violent infantile borderlines" and the process psychotics. At any given time one-third to one-half can be found to function at a marginal level (but with serious residual psychopathology); however, when reassessed several years later many of the individuals appear either better or worse. Although the group percentages are about the same, very few of these individuals maintain consistent adaptive functioning into their early thirties.

Each of the three subgroups of Poor outcome patients is also represented by patients with Adaptive outcomes. Although their numbers are small, their importance is great as future efforts should focus on the attempt to understand these differences in outcome.

Admission Criteria

Clinical folklore supports the value of "early intervention." When faced with unusually difficult patient symptomatology, clinicians often express the wish to have had earlier access to the patient and family, with the belief that treatment techniques used earlier would be more effective. There is some truth to this assertion, but the issue appears to be complex. Treatment techniques need to be matched with the current stage of development of the syndrome. Often there is a sequence: attempting to handle difficulties within the family; reaching out to school personnel, church youth workers or counselors, and primary care physicians; only last seeking specialized professional help. In many cases this is an appropriate natural progression, but in others, it reflects a denial of the severity of the disturbance. Some parents become sensitized to the early recognition of difficulties and move quickly to specialized help. As a consequence, an adolescent involved in disturbed behavior may be referred to a mental health professional before ordinary ways to handle the problems have been fully explored. In rare instances a youngster is referred for inpatient treatment before adequate outpatient treatment has been tried. When there is a poor match between the treatment and the severity of the patient's psychopathology in the direction of overreaction to the youngster's difficulties, not only is the treatment likely to be ineffective, but it also tends to alienate the patient from other forms of treatment that would have been more effective. This problem, although rarely encountered, highlights the importance of developing specific criteria for matching treatment interventions to patient symptoms and behaviors.

Impact of Drug Abuse

In the late 1960s and the early 1970s hospitals were inundated with young people heavily involved in illicit drug abuse. Many clinicians felt that such drug usage is invariably a sign of poor prognosis; this belief persists in some quarters. However, data from our study suggest that use of illicit drugs has little or no prognostic significance in this sample. Illicit drugs are widely available to young people and used to some degree by youngsters across the entire spectrum of psychological functioning, so that the prognostic significance of drug use is insignificant. Measures of severity of psychopathology, clinical estimates of ego strength, and other means of assessing the breadth and depth of psychopathology remain prognostically powerful whether or not a patient has been using drugs.

Following discharge from a psychiatric hospital, many patients return to or begin illicit drug use. With adequate post-discharge psychotherapy, however, the majority soon restrict these activities to social and recreational use of alcohol and marijuana. For a small number who continue heavy polydrug abuse for several years after discharge and resist all the usual forms of treatment, the acceptance of a charismatic (and anti-drug and alcohol) religion or extreme legal pressure (such as a probated felony conviction) may lead to abstinence.

Anger at Hospitalization

Few adolescents present themselves for psychiatric hospital admission in a completely "voluntary" manner. More commonly, adolescents are hospitalized at the request of their parents and/or community authorities. The importance of the patient's anger about hospitalization thus may become a key issue in the establishment of a therapeutic alliance. Lack of staff sensitivity to the depth of rage experienced by many hospitalized patients may impede formation of an effective alliance. Even in a long-term program this anger about hospitalization may continue to surface from time to time and can influence resistance to treatment for months or years. It is impressive to note many years after hospitalization that even those patients who attain Adaptive outcomes often show a continued need to express this incompletely resolved anger. Follow-up interviews suggest at least four sources of anger are present in many patients:

1) The adolescent often experiences his or her hospitalization as profoundly *unfair;* that is, he or she is aware at some level that personal disturbed behaviors reflect (at least in part) family dysfunction for which only the adolescent is hospitalized.
2) Hospitalization is generally experienced by the adolescent as the *loss of a major power struggle* and for many, if not most, adolescents demonstrating severe symptomatic behaviors, power issues within the family are paramount. The youngster's hospitalization is experienced as a victory for others in the family.
3) Compounding the sense of unfairness and loss of control is *separation panic.* This is sometimes manifested directly as severe anxiety, but it is more often reflected (particularly in the adolescent with a personality disorder) as angry, provocative acting out.
4) Finally, underlying these issues (and the last to surface for most youngsters) is a pervasive sense of *guilt* over their own behavior and, in particular, over "failing" their parents.

If these issues are not brought to the surface and worked through, a true treatment alliance may not be possible, and powerful reverberations occur again at the time of discharge when the patient may feel "kicked-out" by an "uncaring" staff. Close examination of problems arising just before discharge may reveal strong elements of a sense of unfairness, a loss of power and control, separation panic, and guilt. Failure to resolve these issues at the time of discharge may diminish the likelihood of maintaining the treatment gains achieved during hospitalizations.

The Patient with Low Intelligence

The frequent finding that youngsters with below-average intelligence do not attain good long-term outcome should not be taken to suggest their being screened out of inpatient treatment programs. Low intelligence does not prevent the formation of a treatment alliance or the occurrence of significant treatment gains in a flexible hospital setting. Many can be treated effectively for their psychiatric dysfunction, but then require special aftercare in order to maintain these gains. The failure to provide adequate, specialized aftercare guidance and support often leads to Poor outcome with patients of lower intellectual capabilities.

Later Major Affective Disorders

Difficulties in accurate diagnosis with adolescents are legion. It is only in recent years, however, that the prevalence of major affective disorders in adolescents has been appreciated. A subgroup of patients followed in this study developed full-blown bipolar syndromes as young adults. Even in retrospect the characteristics that would have identified them as future manic-depressive patients are not clear. Some appeared hyperactive or euphoric, but so did many other adolescents who did not later develop this disorder. Although a few are diagnosed as schizophrenic during adolescence, more often the earlier diagnosis is some variety of personality disorder. As clinical sensitivity to bipolar affective disorder increases, however, youngsters with more classical early signs become obvious. Those who experience excited and expansive behavior alternating with periods of lethargy may warrant a trial on appropriate medication, even if personality disorder symptomatology seems more evident. Carefully obtained family genetic histories may add to early detection of major affective disorders in adolescent patients.

Later Schizophrenic Disorders

Another subgroup of youngsters not originally diagnosed as schizophrenic later develop classical adult schizophrenic syndromes. In the small group of such patients encountered in this study, all were seen originally as severe personality disorders, often with pronounced antisocial features. Unfortunately, differentiation of this subgroup from other severe adolescent personality disorders was not possible. Since there are as yet no psychological or biological signs that invariably precede psychosis, one cannot expect to diagnose all bipolar or schizophrenic patients before a psychotic episode occurs.

Suicide

Suicides in this sample were few, and almost all have been males with severe personality disorders. The depth of internal distress in such youngsters may be obscured by the social distress created by their acting-out behaviors.

Benefits in the Absence of a Treatment Alliance

Although many adolescents with serious personality disorders become actively involved in a treatment alliance during hospitalization, others appear never to form a treatment alliance. They simply manipulate their way through a treatment program. Follow-up contacts with these youngsters and their parents, however, suggest that four forms of gain often are experienced.

1) During the period of hospitalization, such youngsters are removed from many dangers, including drug and alcohol abuse, penal incarceration, physical injury from dangerous acts, pregnancies, and abortions.
2) Hospital peer relationships are often formed around shared interests other than drugs, criminal activities, or other destructive behaviors. These first marginally healthy peer relationships sometimes have later positive impact.
3) Maturation may be greatly accelerated during hospitalization despite the patient's resistance to treatment. This appears to come from more structured living than previously experienced.
4) Tools for future gains may be acquired almost in spite of the patient. Thus the patient learns skills involved in interpersonal relating and in academic or vocational competence which can be utilized when the patient is ready.

Hospital Romances

When adolescents are placed together in an inpatient setting, "hospital romances" occur inevitably. These are often discouraged on the grounds that emotionally disturbed people are not capable of mature love and are not likely to be helpful to each other, or that the intense affects involved divert them from therapeutic goals. Follow-up contacts suggest that staff who resist these liaisons may not only alienate themselves from the youngsters (thus damaging the treatment alliance), but also lose powerful therapeutic leverage. Such romantic involvements may be the first relationships not built on a pathological foundation, and may reflect substantial growth toward healthy relating, however awkward-appearing at the time. The desire to please the loved one often motivates substantial improvements in impulse control, early attempts to work at academic or vocational skills, and other previously unlearned positive behaviors. Although staff may be critical that the improvements occur "for the wrong reasons," follow-up data suggest that the skills and behaviors so acquired may persist long after the "love affair" is over.

Many such relationships last months or even years past hospital discharge, often with considerable mutual benefit. Staff resistance to adolescent patients' romances may convert a potentially therapeutic relationship to a rebellious bonding against authorities. This is reminiscent of their rebellious bonding with peers against their parents, and it effectively prevents the relationships from attaining therapeutic impact—while in some cases prolonging truly disturbed relationships that would "wither away" naturally were they not so arduously opposed.

Peer Relationships

At a somewhat more general level, we have been impressed with both the therapeutic impact and prognostic significance of patient interpersonal relationships. The ability to form and maintain mutually satisfying peer relationships, and the skills involved in attaining peer popularity can easily be underestimated in a treatment program focused on intrapsychic dynamics. It is not uncommon for relationships formed during long-term hospitalization to continue for a number of years. This information suggests that staff attend closely to the number and quality of patients' peer relationships and exert efforts to improve them.

Post-discharge Regression

Some youngsters resume symptomatic behavior shortly after discharge. Anecdotal feedback concerning this tends to lessen staff (and current inpatients') belief in the efficacy of treatment. Post-discharge regression appears to consist of the following elements:

1) Unresolved anger toward parents for hospitalizing them.
2) Unresolved anger at the hospital staff for discharging them.
3) A "sailor-on-the-shore-leave" reaction in which new-found freedoms temporarily overwhelm impulse control.

Those who are not helped to resolve their anger and do not receive adequate psychotherapeutic support may continue their regressive behavior for months or even years, but with adequate preparation for some regression and with continued outpatient therapeutic involvement the majority soon return to their previous higher level of functioning.

Illegitimate Pregnancy

The frequency of illegitimate pregnancy among adolescent and young adult former patients is disconcerting. Providing adequate family life education and contraception techniques needs to be an integral part of both inpatient and aftercare treatment for *all* adolescent patients, regardless of their diagnosis or level of psychopathology.

Charismatic Religion

The attraction of some former patients to fundamentalist, charismatic religions and cults is striking. Some are thought at discharge to be treatment failures, but others make substantial gains. Although it is tempting to explain this attraction only in terms of the continued presence of severe psychopathology, it is our impression that some benefit from their associations with such charismatic religious groups and cults. A few chronically psychotic youngsters attain a degree of belongingness and stability that they are unable to find elsewhere, and some patients with severe personality disorders attain significant periods of impulse control. Most leave these groups within five years or less, although a few individuals remain more religiously oriented than before such membership.

Improved Function in College

Many former adolescent patients seem to function much better academically and socially in college than they did in high school. Obviously this is due in part to therapeutic gain or maturation, but in part it also reflects significant differences between colleges and high schools. Typically, colleges are less rigid and authoritarian in work demands and less intrusive in social rules and regulations. Thus there are fewer areas of conflict for those with unresolved authority problems. In addition, college students typically are allowed a wider variety of "acceptable" social behaviors by their peers than is true among high school peers. Accordingly, it is not wise routinely to advise patients who experience academic and interpersonal difficulties in high school that these will be repeated in a college environment. Some who are never able to manage high school academic, bureaucratic, or social demands are able to function effectively in these areas of college.

FAMILY FINDINGS

Institutional Alliance with Parents

Traditionally, treatment involved separating patients and family members into different treatment situations. Thus, in the old fashioned outpatient clinic or hospital, one mental health professional conducted therapy with the disturbed child, while another member of the treatment team worked with the parental couple, and perhaps a third professional conducted conjoint family sessions. In hospital psychiatry, the focus most often is greater on the hospitalized patient than on the other family members. Admission of an adolescent to a psychiatric hospital, however, is an extreme stress for parents as well. The parents'

intense feelings of loss, guilt, anger, jealousy, fear, and anxiety must
be dealt with effectively if a therapeutic alliance is to be formed.[4] For
most families the greatest crisis points are the periods of hospital admission and discharge, although other crises may occur during the hospital treatment program. In the absence of intensive cognitive and
emotional support, negative parental fantasies may grow and be fueled
by angry or distorted information given them by their hospitalized
adolescent. Although some parents' needs for information and support may seem insatiable, more often this is a reflection of inadequate
staff attention or a treatment philosophy that views parents as alien or
troublesome rather than as integral members of the ongoing treatment
contract and experience.

The hospital's relationship with family members begins before admission of the patient with the reputation or image of the hospital in
the community, but it takes on more concrete character with the first
telephone calls concerning possible admission. From this first contact,
through the time of admission, and until the negotiation of a treatment
plan, most families are in a state of crisis. This period may last for only
a few days, or it may last several weeks, depending on the patient's
needs and on the nature of the institution. However, during this *initial
contact phase* the relationship between family members and hospital
staff revolves around several key issues:

1) Staff gather information from family members concerning a variety
   of patient and family characteristics.
2) Staff and family exchange information concerning the financial
   and administrative portions of their relationships.
3) Staff provide family members with information concerning the
   treatment program's philosophy, procedures, and goals, as well as
   information concerning the patient's day-to-day adaptation to the
   program.
4) Staff provide family members with emotional support and acceptance through frequent personal contacts, the content of which centers around family feelings, questions, factual concerns, or com-
   plaints. This is not a time for confrontations or interpretations if an
   adequate alliance is to be achieved.

Staff avoidance of families during this initial phase exacts a heavy toll later, but frequent contacts focusing on the exchange of information and the provision of support pay many dividends both in treatment process and in long-term outcome.

After staff, patient, and parents have met together in a reporting interview to negotiate an ongoing treatment plan, they may be said to have entered a *working-through phase.* This period may involve several days or many months depending on the nature of the program and the needs of patient and family. During this phase the staff's relationship to the family may shift considerably. Although there is a continuing need to exchange information, more psychologically intensive exploration into marital and family history, dynamics, and current needs may occur. The exact nature of the continuing contact with the family members, however, will depend on the goals and procedures of the negotiated treatment plan. In some cases, information exchange may be the primary continuing relationship, while in others supportive emotional contacts will have high priority. Still other families may be invited to engage in individual psychotherapy, marital therapy, or intensive conjoint family therapy to achieve the agreed-upon goals.

As hospital discharge of the adolescent approaches, the family enters what might be called the *discharge planning and aftercare phase* of the treatment relationship. This phase includes several crucial parts:

1) It is necessary to focus upon specific, concrete details of discharge and aftercare planning. Such details involve arrangements for individual psychotherapy, family therapy, group therapy, medications, or other forms of therapeutic involvement.
2) Special attention is required to prepare for post-discharge role demands—specifically, educational and vocational training, placement, and support. This often overlooked area is perhaps the most significant in terms of impact on long-term level of function.
3) Additional support is required to handle the family members' increased anxiety that predictably occurs immediately before and after discharge of the adolescent.

Time and effort devoted to parents during an adolescent's hospitalization, far from being time taken away from "real" treatment, in fact form the field within which treatment either will or will not take place,

and help determine whether treatment gains persist beyond the patient's discharge.

Family Dysfunction

Independent evaluations of severity of psychopathology of adolescent patients and of their families show significant correlations; that is,
more severely disturbed youngsters tend to come from more severely
dysfunctional families, and youngsters with milder degrees of disturbance tend to come from less dysfunctional families. That knowledge,
however, should not blind clinicians to exceptions. We have seen moderately to profoundly disturbed youngsters in families which, upon
closest scrutiny, do not reveal similar degrees of family dysfunction.
The impact of genetic, neurological, constitutional, or other noninter-
actional variables may produce severe disturbance in a member of a
competent family, just as one often sees relatively healthy siblings in
families with significant dysfunction. Nevertheless, most families of
adolescent inpatients show significant disturbances in the areas of
power, communication, and management of affect which require focused individual, parental, marital, or family therapeutic intervention.

There are three common patterns of family dysfunction seen in the
families of hospitalized adolescents. Because these families are described elsewhere, only a brief summary will be presented here.[1-3]

One pattern involves a dominant-submissive dysfunctional style in
which one parent tightly controls the family. The other parent is much
less powerful and, although often childlike within the family, frequently enters oppositional coalitions with one of the children, particularly the identified adolescent patient. Such families are rigid, oppres-
sive systems and lack affective expressiveness. There is much underlying anger and, often, depression. Although for the most part family
members have clear ego boundaries, they are limited in their range of
humanness and have difficulty separating from the family. Individual
symptomatology commonly emerges when there is developmental
pressure for separation. Although symptomatology can be varied in
quality, most often it is reactive in nature. Acute psychotic reactions,
affective disorders, and severe acting out are common.

A second common dysfunctional pattern is chronic conflict. In this type of family the parents struggle constantly for power, and the children are drawn in—first on one side, then the other. The emotional tone of these families is disagreeable, and open conflict, manipulations, and exploitations are common. Children are apt to leave the family early. A wide range of individual symptomatology is noted, and such families often produce children with severe personality disorders.

The most dysfunctional type of family is that which is chaotic. No family member provides leadership, and the system is characterized by disorganization, aimlessness, and often, severe communication deviance. Many such families avoid active interchange with the surrounding world and maintain an isolated, distrustful orientation. There is an avoidance of change, no push for independence and autonomy, and considerable blurring of individual ego boundaries. It is not surprising that when such family systems produce psychiatric syndromes in their members, the syndromes are severe and often have many process features.

These types of families require different levels of intervention. Resistances to forming an alliance with the hospital staff vary greatly, as does the nature of therapeutic interventions. Some family systems are capable of great change and others appear impervious to all interventions. These factors are often as important for treatment planning as is the nature of the adolescent's psychopathology.

Values Lost and Found

As adolescents move into adulthood, family values that seemed lost or rejected during an adolescent period of rebellion or alienation may reemerge. The young adult may regain such qualities as respectfulness for others, acceptance of responsibility, truthfulness, or other signs of "common decency" long obscured in psychopathology and family conflict, but the reverberations of family system qualities of suspiciousness, cruelty, deceitfulness, or entitlement also may continue. Although treatment interventions around negative family qualities are difficult, opportunities for therapeutic change are not enhanced by therapists' ignoring them and focusing instead upon more easily manageable, concrete behavioral issues.

Parental Abandonment

Working with parents and families for long periods of time may lead the therapist to face the impact upon young patients of withdrawal of parental support in the face of the patient's continued symptomatic state. This withdrawal of support may be augmented by those who emphasize a "sink-or-swim" philosophy at a time during which the patient is patently unable to function and may need more rather than less social support. A review of the subset of former patients who continued marked acting out for many years following the index hospitalization, however, suggests that in many cases persistent parental support, encouragement, and limit-setting, no matter how apparently ineffective, may eventually lead to positive outcome. The complexities of the issue are emphasized by certain instances where parental "abandonment" appears to have a positive impact. It is our impression that such abandonment is most likely to benefit the former patient if the withdrawal of support occurs in a context of anguished giving up, with much exhaustion and sadness and little overt anger. The abandonment process has not proved helpful, however, when the withdrawal of support was an expression of continued scapegoating, lack of true concern, or primarily an angry resolution.

STAFF AND PROGRAM FINDINGS

The Admission Period in Treatment

When asked to evaluate the hospital experience several years after discharge, most former patients touch on crucial aspects of the first day or two of hospitalization. Often these memories are accompanied by strong positive or negative affect. Although descriptions of experiences occurring during the first day or two of hospitalization may represent a kind of "screen memory" or condensation, there is enough factual basis for many of the events described to suggest that staff have an inordinate opportunity to influence the formation of a treatment alliance during the first days of hospitalization. An unusually high level of anxiety renders newly admitted patients sensitive to very small acts of compassion, helpfulness, indifference, or anger. Staff behaviors most often remembered with positive feelings are simple acts of concrete structuring: that is, calm, gentle, unhurried explanations of rules; tours of the unit, school, or other portions of the facility; and assistance with simple matters such as obtaining proper clothing, unpacking, and the other minutiae of moving into a strange environment with new rules, expectations, and procedures.

Staff confrontations concerning patient behavior during the first few days tend to be remembered as extremely intrusive and painful, no matter how gently presented. While this should not be taken to suggest that staff must refrain from confronting all initial negative or destructive patient behavior, it is important to emphasize the unusual impact of staff relationship style at this critical period. Confrontations presented to a new patient in the same fashion that might be helpfully offered several months later may sink like a depth charge, wrecking havoc later in impaired alliance formation.

Helpful Characteristics of Milieu Therapy

Almost every treatment technique described as helpful by some former patients was equally damned by others—restrictions, privileges, individual psychotherapy, off-grounds trips, and family contacts are but a few examples. Any activity, technique, approach, or concept that seems important in the positive development of one patient may be just as severely criticized as harmful or useless by others. This observation is offered to emphasize that dogged adherence to rules, concepts, or procedures may reflect staff rigidity or over-generalization. Procedures found helpful within one group of patients may lose their effectiveness with a different group of patients six months later. An approach to a particular problem that works well for one staff member may backfire when used by another.

Despite the fact that anything remembered as helpful by some patients was recalled by others as harmful, a few generalizations emerge from the follow-up interviews. These include the following:

1) There is increased treatment leverage attained when adolescent patients live together somewhat apart from adult patients and are treat-

ed in a specialized adolescent program involving school as a basic component.

2) Seriously disturbed adolescents require a treatment program with a considerable degree of structure. The degree of structure, however, should vary depending on the level of function of the group and the individual patients who comprise it. Although chaos is never helpful, an egalitarian structure will not function effectively for impulse-ridden adolescent inpatients.

3) The more-or-less constant availability of "someone to talk to" is given a very positive valence by all former patients. Low staff-patient ratios are simply not therapeutically effective.

4) The high degree of oppositionalism present in many adolescent patients tends over time to elicit counter-oppositionalism from even the most dedicated staff. It is through strong team leadership directed toward avoidance of unnecessary power struggles and through an adequate system of interstaff support that constant focus can be maintained on long-term treatment goals.

5) Some organizing "philosophy of treatment" is important. The exact nature of the treatment philosophy appears much less important than the commitment on the part of key staff members to their philosophy. Although it is possible that future collaborative studies examining alternative outcomes of different treatment philosophies may reveal differences, as yet there is no such evidence.

6) When former patients are asked to name and describe those staff persons felt to be most helpful, certain characteristics of effective staff become apparent. These characteristics do *not* include intellectual ability, depth of theoretical knowledge, or years of experience. Rather, effective staff are those who are energetic, highly verbal, and very "warm" in interpersonal style. Although experience, theoretical sophistication, and intelligence may be helpful with adolescent patients, these factors do not carry much therapeutic impact if the person is not *also* energetic, verbal, and warm.

Discharge Criteria

Just as clear criteria for admission to a treatment program need to be evolved, criteria for discharge also need clarification. It is helpful in this regard to view inpatient care as but one phase of the treatment process which should be followed by aftercare tailored to the needs of the individual patient and family. Clear and explicit discharge criteria help responsible staff to maintain constant awareness of the tendency to discharge certain patients prematurely or hold on too long to others, often with unrealistic hopes. While explicit discharge criteria do not remove the necessity of clinical judgment, they do clarify the context within which those judgments may take place.

Individualization of Care

Most treatment programs for adolescents contain mixtures of patients with psychotic and personality disorder syndromes. The particular mix of acute and chronic psychotic disorders and type and severity of personality disorders greatly influences the flavor of a program. Treatment programs that contain a preponderance of psychotic patients will find that treatment techniques appropriate for this group are not best for the severe personality-disordered adolescent. Similarly, programs containing mostly the latter type of patient must modify techniques and approaches if they are to be helpful to overtly psychotic youngsters. Interviews with former patients suggest this may be less a problem with staff on a living unit (nurses, aides, mental health workers), but more a problem in school or other achievement-oriented settings. Demands for sustained attention, tolerance for frustration, "hard work," and productivity tend to elicit very different defensive responses from psychotic and personality-disordered youngsters. For example, the increased staff expectations of adolescents with personality disorders arc often helpful, but they can be overwhelming to the poorly organized psychotic youngsters.

The Special Case

Clinical folklore suggests that "the special case" is a negative process involving staff favoritism of certain patients, leading to a variety of unpleasant consequences. Careful examination of treatment process and outcome of a subgroup of "special case" patients suggests a means of distinguishing positive from negative "special case" treatment planning.

A salient characteristic of all "special case" situations is that key staff members disagree, with some suggesting that the patient "should be treated like everyone else," while others support unusual treatment approaches often involving relief from usual patient obligations. A "special case" does appear to be a destructive procedure when this overt staff disagreement about patient management functions as a smoke screen or displacement for covert staff conflicts. When the overt staff disagreement mostly reflects differences in clinical judgment, much of the negative impact is nullified. Crucial to the success of "special casing" appears to be open staff discussion of their differences concerning the patient and clear communication of these differences to the "special case" patient. When staff are able to discuss their differences with each other and with the patient without undue competitiveness, anger, or covert agenda, "special casing" may lead to very positive treatment outcomes.

Staff Awareness of Prognostic Factors

The importance of completion of inpatient treatment goals and continuation of post-discharge psychotherapy has been emphasized previously. There is a tendency, however, for staff to underutilize this information. Increased staff effort to explain these factors and impress their importance on patients and parents has demonstrated the influence staff may have in persuading unusually difficult patients and families to achieve these goals.

Order of Treatment Impact

Interviewing former patients a number of years after hospitalization has demonstrated a general ordering of those aspects of psychopathology which are affected by treatment.

1) Traditional *symptoms* such as anxiety, depression, and hallucinations are often readily altered in the inpatient setting by the milieu structure, psychotropic medications, and other treatment factors.

2) *Signs* of psychopathology such as impulsivity and poor judgment

are more difficult to influence. With intensive inpatient treatment, however, these also show significant change in a majority of patients.

3) *Relationship skills* appear to require still longer and more intensive work to show long-term changes. In this regard, it should be mentioned that increasing patients' sensitivity to the interactional power of openness, honesty, directness, and sharing of feelings must be balanced by aiding patients to recognize the contexts in which these characteristics are valuable. That is, just as openness, honesty, and detailed sharing of experience may have a profoundly positive impact on intimate relationships, they may be highly inappropriate and self-defeating in other relationships (as, for example, with total strangers, employers, police officers, or personnel directors). When the treatment focus is on utilization of the skills of intimacy, but the importance of context is ignored, discharged patients may fail to match their new skills with the situations in which they find themselves. Upon occasion this may be embarrassing, socially awkward, or otherwise disadvantageous.

4) *Job maintenance skills,* such as dependability, perseverance, suppression of inappropriate affects, and sensitivity to power issues are perhaps the most difficult to alter. Nevertheless, their profound importance demands careful attention and innovative approaches.

Importance of Varied Staff

The therapeutic impact of administrative team leaders and formal psychotherapists (individual, group, and family) is generally well recognized within the hospital. The remaining treatment team members are often described as "ancillary staff." Many former inpatients, however, focus upon very specific benefits received from these "ancillary" personnel and, in fact, not uncommonly attribute major credit to such persons for their most highly valued and lasting gains.

Nurses, aides, and unit mental health workers are most often described as providing the basic security, support, and on-the-spot availability that create a safe environment for growth. School teachers are often described as providing previously unencountered encouragement for the skills of mastery and discipline, and serve as a major source of self-esteem building. Occupational and recreational therapists often receive praise both for teaching specific skills involved in nondestructive ways to obtain pleasure and encouraging creativity.

Frequent references to the positive impact of physical activities and sports are striking. Most adolescent inpatients have had little success with team sports (or any kind of athletics), and not uncommonly refer to improvements in this area as being basic to much personal and interpersonal enjoyment and sense of self-esteem.

It is clear that staff members functioning in a variety of roles in a hospital treatment program often have lasting positive impact on patients. Many patients ascribe equal or greater importance to these staff members than they do to their formal therapists. Programs which underestimate the importance of this finding are sacrificing much of their potential power to influence the patient's growth and development.

REFERENCES

1. Lewis, J. M. *How's Your Family?* New York: Brunner/Mazel, 1979.
2. Lewis, J. M., Beavers, W. R., Gossett, J. T., & Phillips, V. A. *No Single Thread: Psychological Health in Family Systems.* New York: Brunner/Mazel, 1976.
3. Lewis, J. M., Gossett, J. T., & Phillips, V. A. A research study of healthy families. *The Journal of the National Association of Private Psychiatric Hospitals,* 1971, *3* (1), 20–23.
4. Stewart, R. P. Building an alliance between the families of patients and the hospital: Model and process. *The Journal of the National Association of Private Psychiatric Hospitals,* 1981, *12* (2), 63–68.

CHAPTER 10

Treatment Evaluation
in Hospital Psychiatry:
Directions for the Future

Intensive psychiatric hospital treatment is a complex and difficult enterprise. Success requires well-trained, energetic, sensitive staff, willing to persevere in the face of serious patient psychopathology, high cultural expectations, and limited economic support. Severe and often dangerous patient disabilities, finite treatment resources, time pressures, legal concerns, and conflicting theoretical guidelines characterize the field. Staff, patients, and involved family members work together under these trying circumstances to develop positive solutions.

Why add the burden of treatment evaluation? It *is* a burden—it requires personnel, time, and economic support that could be oriented more directly toward treatment itself. We propose that treatment evaluation as an integral part of psychiatric hospital practice is both worthwhile and practical.

RATIONALE

Consumers of mental health services deserve the finest quality care that can be provided, delivered in the most efficient manner possible. The professionals involved in delivering such services cannot know the degree to which they approach maximum effectiveness and efficiency unless they develop a systematic approach to the evaluation of the treatment program.

Intuitive, theoretical and, in some cases, empirical hypotheses concerning the effects of particular treatment techniques, approaches, and programs guide the day-to-day decisions of psychiatric hospital staff. Without clear, scientific feedback concerning the effectiveness of various techniques and approaches, clinicians are engaged in a blindfolded practice that does not provide the corrections and improvements necessary to plan treatment with greater helpfulness and efficiency.

Well designed quality assessment creates a treatment-modifying feedback loop that moves the hospital system toward increasing treatment successes and decreasing failure. We are beyond the question of whether or not psychiatric hospital treatment helps, just as we are beyond the question of whether psychotherapy helps.[16] Rather, research can be directed more profitably toward establishing which treatment approaches, and under what circumstances, are most beneficial for various kinds of patients. Studies debating the usefulness of short-term versus long-term inpatient care, inpatient versus day hospital treatment, or the use of psychotherapy versus medications, although timely in the past, may be seen currently as steps toward more integrated research which will strive to identify the most beneficial matching of treatment approaches with identifiable patient needs.

It is likely, for example, that many psychological problems are resolved without formal treatment through reliance on family and friends, the passage of time, and planned or fortuitous changes in life circumstances. More chronic or serious problems may require the help available from general physicians, clergy, or mental health professionals engaged in outpatient counseling and psychotherapy. In still more severe difficulties, considerations of day hospital and inpatient treatment arise. At this point it is particularly clear that empirically based guidelines do not exist: What are the proper indications for outpatient psychotherapy, medications, partial hospitalization, short-term inpatient treatment, and long-term inpatient care? What types of patients, family support systems, diagnostic groupings or personality conflicts are more efficiently and effectively treated with these approaches? While mental health professionals may have educated guesses about such vital issues, we all will be more able to match optimal treatment programs to patients' needs only when we establish assessment research as a basic component to all treatment programs.

In addition, treatment evaluation can perform a crucial function in psychiatric hospitals by its positive effects on staff morale. Because treatment failures do occur despite maximum effort, the sustaining and invigorating effect of documented successes is extremely important. Anecdotal feedback about former patients after hospital discharge is almost invariably "bad news." When an ex-patient commits suicide, returns to alcohol or drug abuse, or attains notoriety through destructive actions, the news reverberates quickly through hospital staff. On the other hand, patients who leave the treatment setting, make a success of their intimate relationships, perform their work adequately, and have no further need of mental health contacts generally disappear from the view of the hospital staff. Thus, over a period of years, morale can grind down, and sometimes even faith in the efficacy of treatment programs can be lost. Systematic treatment assessment research, however, indicates very substantial rates of improvement, both short- and long-term. In a field where most of what we do is mediated through day-to-day interpersonal contacts between patients, their family members, and hospital staff, front-line treatment personnel are sustained and invigorated by realizing their therapeutic influence.

Hospital treatment programs are under great pressure for accountability from the general public, from insurance carriers, from professional organizations, and from government agencies. As individuals become more sophisticated, they demand proof that health care is being delivered in the highest quality possible and with maximum efficiency. Insurance carriers are deeply invested in both quality assurance and cost containment. The development of Professional Standards Review Organizations (PSROs) creates additional needs for hospital staff to justify admissions, continuation of treatment beyond very brief periods, and detailed discharge planning. PSROs also require that hospitals document the quality and utilization of their services on an ongoing and scheduled basis. The Joint Commission on Accreditation of Hospitals provides highly detailed guidance in its Consolidated Standards, assuring maximum quality and efficiency.[2] Government agencies at all levels have come to require integrated program evaluation on the part of any health care delivery system supported by government funds.

For these reasons, treatment evaluation must become a basic component of all psychiatric hospital treatment programs. There are several worthwhile approaches to such treatment evaluation. At the most basic level, treatment evaluation consists of strengthening *clinical* approaches to assessment: individual case review, medical and nursing audit, utilization review, and other quality assurance activities.[2] Individual case review involves periodic reexamination of each patient's treatment plan, with sharing and consultation concerning progress and problems by all members of the patient's treatment team, and including consultations from other clinical staff not so immediately involved in the patient's treatment. Medical and nursing audits involve the systematic examination of discharged and current patients' medical records to evaluate the degree to which various aspects of the treatment plan conform to established criteria. The process of utilization review, which also relies upon predefined criteria, evaluates the match between patients' needs and hospital treatment resources, insuring that treatment services are necessary, economically efficient, and effective. Because these activities are required for Joint Commission accreditation, they are found in most psychiatric hospitals. They vary widely, however, in the degree of their integration, the status they hold within a treatment institution, the amount of personnel time and effort provided, and the degree of respect given to their findings. Improved treatment evaluation logically begins with strengthening these required approaches in a comprehensive quality assurance plan.

A second step toward more adequate treatment evaluation is that of implementing *short-term and sharply focused research evaluation studies.* Their content will often reflect the immediate needs and interests of concerned staff: evaluation of professional training programs (such as those for psychiatric residents, psychology interns, or psychiatric nursing students); development of a staff-peer evaluation system; examination of advantages and disadvantages of different ways of charting medical records; assessment of the immediate efficacy of using different patterns of various treatments (individual, group, and family psychotherapy, medications, and occupational or recreational activities); comparison of the immediate effects of different treatment team styles; comparison of psychotropic medications; development of pre-treatment and post-treatment evaluation measures for various programs; ongoing evaluation, consultation, and feedback during the development of new treatments; studies of treatment for special populations (age or diagnostic groups); studies of the salient characteristics of differing treatment team milieus; or other studies growing out of a particular need of a particular hospital's clinical and administrative staff.

Finally, at a third level, the sine qua non of hospital treatment evaluation is the *long-term outcome follow-up study*. It might seem at first glance that if the ultimate goal is treatment evaluation, adequate results could be obtained by measuring the course of patient change from the time of hospital admission to the time of discharge, without relying upon more difficult and time-consuming follow-up contacts. Erickson demonstrates the fallacy of that approach, however, in his exhaustive review of adult psychiatric hospital evaluation studies.[4] After examining a number of studies that demonstrate significant degrees of patient improvement, Erickson summarizes,

> But given the data we have, it is tempting to conclude that practically any reasonable innovation will lead to improvement.

That is, 65–75 percent improvement rates *during hospitalization* are frequently noted, almost without regard to the type or severity of patient psychopathology, the duration of the hospital treatment, the nature of the treatment program, or the methods of defining or assessing improvement.

After exploring criticisms of these studies, Erickson indicates,

> However, attacks on the internal validity of inhospital studies are of less significance than the pressing question, Do improvements shown in hospital settings persist? On the one hand, it may be true that given adequate time, patients *as a group* are restored to premorbid functioning in the hospital, and this improvement persists

over a reasonable follow-up period. . . . But the disheartening
and repeated finding is that measures taken in the hospital are not
correlated with posthospital adjustment. . . .

Those who show good adjustment in the hospital are not necessarily the same individuals who will show good adjustment in the
community later on. In the final analysis the question is not How
fast was the patient discharged? or How well did he do in the hospital? but What served to restore or improve his psychological
functioning in the community following discharge (p. 529)?[4]

In his review of hospital treatment research, Ellsworth noted,

It matters little if the client learns to adjust well to the hospital setting or in relating to his clinic therapist if his behavior at work or
his relationship to family members is not satisfactory. A basic assumption made by many mental health professionals has been that
a client's adjustment and behavior in the treatment setting is highly related to his adjustment in other settings. This assumption is
not correct, for patients often behave quite differently in treatment settings than they do in community settings. . . . The measures of program effectiveness that deserve most attention, then,
are measures of clients' behavior in the community setting (p.
240-241).[3]

Both Erickson[4] and Ellsworth[3] refer to a series of studies that consistently demonstrate very low, nonsignificant correlations between in-
hospital improvements and levels of function with later posthospital
behavioral improvements and levels of function.

Patients do not arrive at hospitals in order to be helped to function
more adequately in hospitals. On the contrary, they arrive with hopes
that they will demonstrate improved levels of personal, social, and vocational functioning in their home community following discharge.
Accordingly, adequate psychiatric hospital evaluation studies must include examination of patients' posthospital levels of function in significant life areas.

It is beyond the scope of this book to provide a detailed presentation
of the technical issues involved in hospital follow-up assessment, and

we have addressed these issues elsewhere.[6,8] It is our belief that follow-up research can be tailored to the organizational structure and goals of each treatment institution, and an appropriate form of systematic, objective, and comprehensive follow-up treatment assessment can be made a basic part of every psychiatric hospital's treatment program. This explication of general issues encountered in such programs is intended to help others approach these tasks more efficiently and effectively.

PROBLEMS

Certain problems and conflicts tend to occur in all forms of treatment evaluation, whether one is strengthening mandated hospital quality assurance committees, developing short-term focused research projects, or initiating long-term follow-up. In our experience, these difficulties tend to be most severe, however, with regard to long-term outcome.

The ultimate goal of the hospital staff is to assist patients and their families achieve adaptive posthospital functioning. Therefore, the long-term follow-up study provides the clearest evidence of the staff's effectiveness. The problems and conflicts encountered in this task will be presented in four primary areas: measurement issues, design issues, clinical issues, and hospital system issues. Techniques for dealing with these problems and conflicts are offered in the hope of encouraging other treatment institutions to inaugurate long-term follow-up studies.

Measurement Issues

Hospital staff devote themselves to patient "improvement"; their desire is that after discharge the patient will operate at a higher "level of function." What is meant by "improvement" and "level of function"? In their work on psychotherapy assessment, Strupp, Hadley, and Gomez-Schwartz stress the importance of considering different perspectives of treatment outcome.[15] They describe a tripartite model and explain it as follows:

Three major interested parties are concerned with definitions of
mental health: (1) *society* (including significant persons in the patient's life); (2) the *individual patient;* and (3) the *mental health
professional.* Each of these parties defines mental health in terms
of certain unique purposes or aims it seeks to fulfill and conse-
quently, each focuses on specific aspects of an individual's functioning in determining his mental health.

1. *Society* is primarily concerned with the maintenance of social
relations, institutions, and prevailing standards of sanctioned
conduct. Society and its agents thus tend to define mental health
in terms of behavioral stability, predictability, and conformity to
the social code. . . .

2. The *individual client,* evaluating his own mental health uses a
criterion distinctly different from that used by society. The individual wishes first and foremost to be happy, to feel content. He
defines mental health in terms of highly subjective feelings of well
being—feelings with a validity all their own . . .

3. Most *mental health professionals* tend to view an individual's
functioning within the framework of some theory of personality
structure which transcends social adaptation and subjective well
being . . . (p. 94–96).[15]

Strupp et al. indicate that psychotherapy resulting in improvement
(or deterioration) from any single point of view may or may not be accompanied by similar changes from the other vantage points.

We suggest that the third area, definition of patient change in terms
of conformity to some theory of personality, is the least important in
hospital psychiatry. Changes noted on psychological tests or thought
to have taken place at some psychodynamic level are not considered to
be significant unless they are accompanied by improvements either in
the individual's subjective feeling state or in clearly identifiable behavioral changes.

Probably few patients are admitted to a psychiatric hospital primarily because of unpleasant internal feeling states. Hospital treatment,
whether sought voluntarily by the patient or at the behest of others,
generally takes place because the patient's overt behavior is either de-
monstrably dangerous or severely self-defeating. These characteristics

are virtually universal among those admitted to inpatient care. Patients vary widely, however, in the degree to which they experience themselves and their life situations as either happy or distressing.

In evaluating psychiatric hospital care, the primary criteria at follow-up should be those based upon observable interpersonal, vocational, and symptomatic behaviors that promote successful functioning in the outside world. For the purpose of evaluating hospital treatment, the ways in which patients feel about themselves and their treatment experience, while of great meaning, are less important than the practical quality of their posthospital adjustment. This, of course, is the authors' value judgment about what changes "should" be seen as the result of treatment.

The issue of patients' level of function after discharge raises the question of whose judgments should be sought: staff, former patients, or close family members? We feel that the best assessment of treatment outcome derives from independent judgments of professionals and is based on the current level of the patient's interpersonal, vocational, and symptomatic function as reported by *both* the former patient and the closest family member, usually a spouse or parent, who was involved with the patient both at the time of admission and at the time of follow-up.

In summary, research staff can design questionnaires and interview schedules, gather follow-up data, and render professional judgments of levels of function, but these judgments should be heavily influenced by a focus upon concrete behavioral signs of interpersonal, occupational, and symptomatic behaviors exhibited by the former patient and described both by that individual and the closest family member.

Next, then, is the question of how best to obtain follow-up information: psychological tests, standardized scales, questionnaires, face-to-face interviews, or telephone contacts? From the previous discussion it is clear that we do not feel that current standardized psychological tests are very helpful in follow-up assessment, but this should not preclude continued attempts to find relevant test indices of hospital treatment impact. Face-to-face interviews provide maximum information, but are prohibitively expensive in personnel time if attempted on every former patient and significant family member. Mailed questionnaires and rating scales may be useful, although they produce significant

168   To Find a Way

problems of data loss and inevitable bias in the results. Telephone contacts offer a compromise between the data loss of questionnaires and
scales and the expense of face-to-face interviews. Combining assessment approaches, depending upon the specific circumstances of a giv-
en institution, is in our judgment the most reasonable approach.

In previous chapters we note the tendency of measures of psychopathology to be highly effective in predicting adaptive outcome, but
much less effective for adequate prediction of poor outcome. Improving such measures would help, but in addition, there is a need for new,
practical means of assessing patients' ego strengths. Reliable measures
of ego strength, competence, or adaptability may very well predict more
accurately those patients displaying severe psychopathology who, following treatment, will be able to function well in society.

The researchers' ability to reflect clinical complexities in multivariate measurement can be augmented by careful development of patient,
family, treatment process, and outcome measures before beginning
data collection. Although the field is still evolving, sufficient work has
now been accomplished to make this approach a realistic possibility.

Design Issues

Few mental health professionals are trained to conduct treatment
evaluation research. Those with research training have most often
been taught elegant designs in which the researchers must obtain maximum control over the experimental conditions, applying methodological strategies aimed at holding many variables constant or canceling
them through random assignment. This ideal controlled experimental
model leads to great confidence that differences in the subsequent behavior of the experimental and control groups are a function of their
exposure to the treatment condition. Unfortunately, this design does
not lend itself to the practical realities of hospital treatment programs,
except in some instances of drug comparison studies. Summarizing
these problems, Ellsworth notes:

In many program evaluation studies, one is not only unable to
control all the relevant treatment variables and to assign patients

in random fashion, but one faces such problems as data loss. This is especially troublesome when follow-up data are collected after the patient has left the treatment setting. In order to avoid this, most program evaluators collect data while the patient remains in the treatment setting. But, as already seen, these data are not adequate if one wishes to know something about the program's effect on the patient's behavior in other settings. Faced with these kinds of problems, program evaluation is more like that of introducing a sophisticated information system rather than implementing an experimental study. And program evaluation becomes increasingly scientific as one designs his study so as to minimize the possibility that outcome differences are a function of such uncontrolled factors as population differences, differential data loss, and the like (p. 256–257).[3]

Fortunately, worthwhile approaches to treatment evaluation are available even though true experimental designs rarely can be used. It is not the purpose of this book to instruct in the fundamentals of design of treatment outcome studies. A recent increase in interest in treatment evaluation, however, makes such information readily available.[1,5,7,14] For our purposes it is sufficient to say that the variety of technical design problems encountered by any potential investigator can be met in ways that allow evaluation studies to proceed to practical and useful conclusions.

Clinical Issues

Quite apart from the technicalities of design and methodology, there is a commonsense problem that plagues any follow-up researcher: demonstrating that changes noted at the time of follow-up exceed those which might have taken place in an unassisted maturation. This is the problem of "spontaneous remission"—how can it be known patients wouldn't have improved just as much without treatment? Ideally, one would wish to have persons with equivalent psychological dysfunction assigned randomly to treatment and no-treatment groups. While this has been accomplished at times in outpatient psychotherapy, it is more difficult to accomplish with those who, because of dangerous or destructive behavior, need inpatient care. In his critical review of outpatient psychotherapy studies, Parloff concludes,

> A review of controlled studies permits the conclusion that psychodynamic therapies, client-centered psychotherapy, cognitive therapies, and behavioral therapies have achieved results that are superior to no-treatment procedures. The findings based on diverse studies using diverse criteria, offer an affirmative global answer to the question of whether psychotherapies are more effective than spontaneous remission rates. . . .[11]

Another review summarized nearly 700 published and unpublished psychotherapy studies, each of which included an untreated control group.[13] This permits an estimate of relevant rates of spontaneous recovery in each study. In over 90 percent of the experiments, the psychotherapy group improved more than the control group. Also, the median person receiving psychotherapy was better off than 80 percent of the untreated controls. Because of practical, ethical, humanitarian, and legal concerns, comparable studies of inpatient populations are virtually nonexistent. However, certain findings reviewed by Erikson bear on this issue.[4]

A standard experimental approach to assessing the impact of a given intervention when a nontreatment control group is impossible is to compare the impact of providing different levels or intensities of the intervention program. Thus, for example, in a series of studies, Erikson notes different outcome levels depending upon such factors as hospital size and staff-patient ratios in the treating institutions. Smaller hospitals have higher rates of treatment success than larger ones, and hospitals with higher staff-patient ratios have better patient outcome than those with lower staff-patient ratios. Factors such as increased emphasis on family-care programs also improve treatment outcome. While these studies are correlational in nature and thus do not *prove* that the variables being measured necessarily cause the outcomes noted, they are nevertheless consistent with the interpretation.

Other studies reviewed by Erikson demonstrate that in large hospital settings randomly selected patients exposed to various special treatment programs tend to do better than those in control groups who did not receive special programs. This suggests that merely being hospitalized does little to help profoundly disturbed individuals, but that active, intensive, and well-designed treatment programs produce demonstrable patient improvement and that the levels of improvement correlate well with the amount of intensive, organized treatment. A more recent review of research on psychotherapy outcome with adolescents, both outpatient and inpatient, presents essentially similar conclusions.[16] The bulk of evidence suggests that both inpatient and outpatient treatment are capable of producing positive changes over and above that which would take place without treatment, if the services provided are of sound quality.

The few available studies of disturbed but untreated adolescents point out that spontaneous remission of moderate-to-severe adolescent psychopathology is much less common than what might be called "spontaneous deterioration." Symptomatic adolescents tend, by and large, to become symptomatic adults.[9,12,17] In addition, the observation that most patients referred for long-term intensive care have already progressed through a series of increasingly intense treatment services with no lasting results suggests more of a trend toward continuing disturbance than spontaneous recovery.

Studies of well-functioning, untreated adolescents, as summarized recently by Oldham, demonstrate clearly that normal teenagers do not show the types of severe behavioral disturbances seen in clinical populations.[10] Adolescents who act disturbed *are* disturbed—they are not merely passing through "adolescent turmoil"—and should not be expected to outgrow their difficulties without assistance.

The evidence, then, suggests that severe disturbances are better treated than left alone and that intensive hospital treatment is more effective than custodial care for seriously disturbed individuals. There remains the question of whether the changes noted are due primarily to the treatment itself or to a "placebo effect," derived from suggestion, expectations, and attention. Studies of the "placebo effect" are, of course, important when one is evaluating the impact of a new medication. In order to demonstrate the effectiveness of a given drug on certain symptoms, one must be able to subtract from the effectiveness that change which would have taken place if the patient had been given an inert substance but led to believe that the substance was an effective medication. The analogy becomes quite strained, however, when applied to psychiatric hospital treatment, much of which consists of institutional structure, empathic understanding, clear communications, interpretations, and the provision of hope. Are these characteristics "placebo," or are they an integral part of effective psychiatric hospital practice? Perhaps there is no truly "inert" human interaction; human relationships, whether in a hospital or out, always produce effects for better or worse. Again quoting Parloff's review of outpatient psychotherapy research,

> However, such literature as is available does suggest that treatment effects are usually more powerful than those found in the placebo control group. . . . The review of psychotherapy research summarized by Glass and Smith . . . concluded that the placebo effect was less than half as large as the effects of the other elements in the psychotherapy relationship.[11]

Our inability at this time to specify exactly which treatment variables are most powerful with varying patient groups does not minimize the positive effects obtained. Rather, this problem should stimulate investigators to conduct more discriminating comparison studies wherever possible.[16]

Hospital System Issues

When one begins to conduct treatment evaluation research in a hospital setting, some staff objections may be encountered. In our judgment, these objections on the part of clinical and administrative staff should not be dismissed as neurotic "resistance," but rather, respected and dealt with openly, thereby substantially improving the eventual success of treatment evaluation efforts.[6,8]

Clinicians and administrators may object to the institution of treatment evaluation because they fear that poorly conducted studies which they cannot direct or supervise (nor, in some cases, completely understand) may demonstrate that the treatment being provided is ineffective. Much of what mental health professionals do occurs through the medium of personal interaction, and if the results are disappointing, the indictment may be felt as unusually intense and personal. When a researcher ignores this fear or treats it as a manifestation of neurosis, unwarranted defensiveness, or professional incompetence, the resistance escalates. But a very different climate can be created if the researcher appreciates the power and reality of this fear and encourages open exploration of the details of the project, with assurance that it is directed toward improving everyone's therapeutic impact.

Clinicians and administrators may fear research personnel if they sense that the researchers are ignorant of the primacy of clinical needs and procedures. For this reason, the research is facilitated when those so engaged are themselves clinicians and, if possible, are involved in clinical work concurrent with their research activities.

Clinical decision-makers may object to evaluation research on the grounds that it will interfere with their ability to decide clinical issues. This objection clearly requires a delicate negotiation of the role of the researchers within the clinical setting. Too much power to influence clinical decisions will prove counterproductive to the evaluation research, just as too little power may undermine the process of evaluation. Open negotiation of this issue is to be preferred over ignoring it or handling it indirectly. The effective conduct of a treatment evaluation study is greatly augmented if the research has maximum support from the highest levels of power within the hospital system. The researcher must have this support from the top in order to negotiate effectively with important clinical and administrative personnel about the various system issues being described.

The evaluation researcher needs to anticipate spending what may seem an inordinate amount of time explaining the procedures, goals, and potential for staff growth of the evaluation study. If this is done at first, then clinical staff enthusiasm and participation will be more readily forthcoming. Repeated focus on the specific procedures to be followed, emphasis on the means by which patient and staff confidentiality and anonymity are to be protected, and frequent demonstrations by word and deed of respect for patients and staff concerns will reassure anxieties and elicit cooperation.

The nature of treatment outcome work is such that one often cannot provide instant feedback, but it is imperative (and also relatively easy) to develop ways to give something for every imposition the research requires. Simply telling hospital staff that a project will provide them with clinically useful information, however, is not sufficient. An attitude of reciprocity may be expressed by systematically providing copies of recent journal articles on topics of immediate relevance to patient care or making certain aspects of data collection readily available to clinicians, even if the data are not in final form. A periodic "in-house" progress report requires little work and often is helpful to researchers in organizing preliminary findings. Failure to provide such feedback is self-defeating, especially in projects that continue for long periods of time. Treatment personnel who learn that their time is being taken with nothing given in return will understandably "resist" continued participation.

The use of deception in clinical research is almost always destructive and rarely, if ever, necessary. For example, a frequent research strategy is to tell research subjects that one is measuring variable A, when, in fact, variable B is being measured. Reliance on such deceptive techniques in research evaluation projects will lead to a level of distrust that will cause the projects substantial grief at a later point in time. We remain unaware of any relevant treatment evaluation questions that require a deceptive research approach.

Finally, hospital personnel may object to evaluation research on the ground that it takes too much of their time to fill out forms and make observations. This objection can be largely defused by never asking a clinician to do anything that a researcher can do. If there are observations to be made that research staff can make, or that can be made by a student, a professional trainee, or other observer, then it is best not to ask a member of the clinical staff to make these observations. Effort devoted to minimizing the time required of treatment staff in data collection is well invested. Some ratings, judgments, or other data can be provided only by a psychotherapist, a hospital psychiatrist, or a nurse, and in these cases cooperation is enhanced when clinical staff are aware that their time is highly valued. They are also more likely to cooperate if fully informed of the nature of the project, if impressed with the potential clinical value of the findings, and if appropriately included in deciding relevant project issues.

In summary, we believe treatment evaluation is a necessary and helpful component of psychiatric hospital treatment. We suggest three levels of involvement in treatment evaluation: strengthening of quality assurance activities; introducing short-term focused projects; and finally, developing long-term outcome follow-up studies. We believe these form the basis for a comprehensive approach to the assurance of highest quality and maximum efficiency in psychiatric hospital treatment.

REFERENCES

1. Anderson, S. B., & Ball, S. *The Profession and Practice of Program Evaluation.* San Francisco: Josey-Bass, 1978.
2. *Consolidated Standards Manual for Child, Adolescent, and Adult Psychiatric, Alcoholism, and Drug Abuse Facilities.* Chicago: Joint Commission on Accrediation of Hospitals, 1981.
3. Ellsworth, R. B. Consumer feedback in measuring the effectiveness of mental health programs. In M. Guttentag & E. L. Struening (Eds.), *Handbook of Evaluation Research,* Vol. II. Beverly Hills: Sage Publications, 1975, pp. 239-274.
4. Erickson, R. C. Outcome studies in mental hospitals: A review. *Psychological Bulletin,* 1975, *82,* 519-540.
5. Franklin, J. L., & Thrasher, J. H. *An Introduction to Program Evaluation.* New York: John Wiley & Sons, 1976.
6. Gossett, J. T. Guidelines for research in a clinical setting. *Journal of the National Association of Private Psychiatric Hospitals,* 1978, *10* (2), 19-27.
7. Guttentag, M., & Struening, E. L. (Eds.) *Handbook of Evaluation Research,* Vol. II. Beverly Hills: Sage Publications, 1975.
8. Lewis, S. B., Barnhart, F. D., Gossett, J. T., & Phillips, V. A. Follow-up of adolescents treated in a psychiatric hospital: Operational solutions to some methodological problems of clinical research. *American Journal of Orthopsychiatry,* 1975, *45* (5), 813-824.
9. Masterson. J. The symptomatic adolescent five years later: He didn't grow out of it. *American Journal of Psychiatry,* 1967, *123,* 1338-1345.
10. Oldham, D. G. Adolescent turmoil: A myth revisited. In S. C. Feinstein & P. L. Giovacchini (Eds.), *Adolescent Psychiatry,* Vol. 6. Chicago: University of Chicago Press, 1978.
11. Parloff, M. B. Can psychotherapy research guide the policymaker: A little knowledge may be a dangerous thing. *American Psychologist,* 1979, *34,* 296-306.
12. Robins, L. N. *Deviant Children Grown Up.* Baltimore: Williams and Wilkins, 1966.
13. Smith, M. L., & Glass, G. V. Meta-analysis of psychotherapy outcome studies. *American Psychologist,* 1977, *32*(9), 752-760.
14. Stromsdorfer, E. W., & Farkas, G. (Eds.) *Evaluation Studies Review Annual,* Vol. 5. Beverly Hills: Sage Publications, 1980.

15. Strupp, H. H., Hadley, S. W., & Gomez-Schwartz, B. *Psychotherapy for Better or Worse.* New York: Jason Aronson, 1977.
16. Tramontana, M. G. Critical review of research on psychotherapy outcome with adolescents: 1967–1977. *Psychological Bulletin,* 1980, *88* (2), 429–450.
17. Weiner, S., & DelGaudio, A. Psychopathology in adolescence. *Archives of General Psychiatry,* 1976, *33,* 187–193.

APPENDIX A

Gossett-Timberlawn Adolescent Psychopathology Scale

Total Score _____

Patient _____

Date ,_____

Rater _____

Psychiatric Hospital Admission Form: Based on everything you know about this patient, evaluate his or her level of functioning during the most characteristic weeks or months just prior to hospital admission.

How well do you know this patient?

Discussion: The knowledge scale is an opportunity for you to indicate the confidence you have concerning rating the adolescent. We are not referring to the confidence of choosing alternative 16 over 14, but rather your ability to substantiate your choice based on personal observation of the adolescent. Choosing alternative 1 on this scale would mean that you could substantiate most, if not all, of your ratings based on personal observation.

_____ 1. I know this adolescent extremely well.

_____ 2.

_____ 3. I know this adolescent fairly well.

_____ 4.

_____ 5. I do not know this adolescent well.

_____ 6.

_____ 7. I do not know this adolescent.

Note: Please do not add your responses to this scale to your total psychopathology score.

I. *Autonomy: The person's ability to function independently vs. need to be protected and/or supported by a therapist or hospital.*

_____   1. Productive autonomy; superior adaptation at an independent level.

_____   2.

_____   3. Normal, average, healthy level of genuine autonomy.

_____   4.

_____   5. Still within the "normal" range, but occasional or mild reliance on alcohol, tranquilizers (or other prescribed or self-medication), or other basically normal regulatory devices to maintain functioning.

_____   6.

_____   7. Need for outpatient psychotherapy (or equivalent) in order to function.

_____   8.

_____   9. Possible need for inpatient management; need a more extended period of evaluation to determine whether needs outpatient or inpatient management.

_____ 10.

_____ 11. Clear need for inpatient management but expect this person to have little difficulty in rapidly earning or maintaining grounds privilege status.

_____ 12.

_____ 13. Clear need for inpatient management and expect this person to have moderate difficulty in earning or maintaining grounds privilege status.

_____ 14.

_____ 15. Clear need for inpatient management and expect this person to be unable to leave a locked unit, unless accompanied, for an extended period of time.

_____ 16.

_____ 17. Clear need for inpatient management and expect this person to be unable to leave a locked unit for an extended period of time.

_____ 18.

_____ 19. Need for constant inpatient supervision and control such as special duty nursing care or physical restraint.

II. *Diagnostic Severity: The degree of personality integration or disorganization in psychodiagnostic terms.*

_____   1. Superior level of personality integration and organization.

_____   2.

_____ 3. Average, everyday, healthy level of personality integration and organization.

_____ 4.

_____ 5. While still essentially normal, slight but definite disturbance of organization; slight, but definite impairment of smooth adaptive control—"nervousness."

_____ 6.

_____ 7. More than everyday discomfort resulting from a substantial amount of energy being harnessed by mildly neurotic tension-reducing and compensating living devices. No personality or psychotic symptoms noted.

_____ 8.

_____ 9. Clear mild neurotic symptoms, inhibitions, or mechanisms are noted, but in addition, there is a suggestion of some possible personality defects or disturbances.

_____ 10.

_____ 11. Moderate neurotic disorder _or_ a clear mild personality disorder; behaviors may include (but are not limited to) fainting spells, phobias, psychosomatic reactions, drug abuse, suicide gestures, rituals, sexual deviances, generalized inadequacy, exaggerated passivity or aggressiveness, and so forth.

_____ 12.

_____ 13. Severe neurotic disorder, _or_ moderate personality disorder, _or_ hints of mild compensated or underlying psychosis; behaviors here may be similar to #11 above, but are seen as more frequent, more constant, or more severe.

_____ 14.

_____ 15. Profound neurotic disorder, _or_ severe personality disorder, _or_ clear borderline and mild to moderate overt psychotic disorder; behaviors here may include (but are not limited to) chronic repetitive violent aggression, expansive and excited syndromes, episodic violence, near total dysfunction due to extreme withdrawal, or phobic or severely passive life style, etc.

_____ 16.

_____ 17. Profound personality disorder _or_ servere overt psychosis; behaviors here may include (but are not limited to) severe addictive states, extreme states of disorganization, regression, and reality repudiation as in delirium, severe paranoid or depressed psychoses, confusion, catatonia, etc.

_____ 18.

_____ 19. Malignant anxiety and depression which, if not immediately controlled by external devices will eventuate in death; psychogenic death, psychotic depressive suicide; total despair, ego disintegration and exhaustion.

III. *Subjective Discomfort: The degree of distress consciously experienced by the individual while engaged in age-appropriate scholastic, vocational, and interpersonal situations. If the person generally avoids such situations through running away, passivity, or other avoidance style defenses (denial, repression, etc.), rate the degree of discomfort you judge the person would feel in age-appropriate school, work, or interpersonal situations if the avoidance mechanisms were suddenly removed.*

_____ 1. Unusual degree of serenity based on superior personality organization.

_____ 2.

_____ 3. Average, everyday, healthy level of experienced comfort.

_____ 4.

_____ 5. Vague or occasional discomfort; mild anxiety, worry, restlessness, or somatic dysfunction.

_____ 6.

_____ 7. Clear occasional discomfort of a mild degree; anxiety, depression, or somatization; this degree of discomfort will sometimes motivate the person to seek religious, medical, psychotherapeutic, self-medicated, or other tension-reducing aid.

_____ 8.

_____ 9. Clear frequent discomfort of a mild degree; anxiety, depression, somatization, loneliness, or negative feedback elicited by one's behavior; this degree of discomfort will sometimes motivate the person to seek religious, medical, psychotherapeutic, self-medicated, or other tension-reducing aid.

_____ 10.

_____ 11. Occasional discomfort of a moderate degree from symptoms or environmental feedback; may be some brief episodes of extreme discomfort; this degree of discomfort will usually motivate the person to seek religious, medical, psychotherapeutic, self-medicated, or other tension-reducing aid.

_____ 12.

_____ 13. Frequent or continuous moderate discomfort from symptoms or environmental feedback; may be some brief episodes of extreme discomfort; this degree of discomfort will usually motivate the person to seek religious, medical, psychotherapeutic, self-medicated, or other tension-reducing aid.

_____ 14.

_____ 15. Severe symptom discomfort; frequent intense discomfort from extreme anxiety attacks, depressions, psychophysiological symptoms or negative environmental feedback; this degree of discomfort will almost invariably motivate the person to seek religious, medical, psychotherapeutic, self-medicated, or other tension-reducing aid.

_____ 16.

_____ 17. Severe symptom discomfort; continuous intense discomfort from extreme anxiety attacks, depressions, psychophysiological symptoms or negative environmental feedback; this degree of discomfort will almost invariably motivate the person to seek religious, medical, psychotherapeutic, self-medicated, or other tension-reducing aid.

_____ 18.

_____ 19. Profound symptom discomfort; continuous and extreme discomfort as in panic, delirium, utter helpless/hopelessness; person may seek some kind of tension-reducing aid or may be unable to do so.

IV. _Environmental Effect: The manner in which the person's behavior influences those around him; rate according to how an "average person" would judge the situation._

_____ 1. Superior positive effect on family, peers, school or community through unusual productivity, leadership, or participation.

_____ 2.

_____ 3. Average, everyday, healthy effect on others; not remarkably constructive or destructive with family, peers, school or community.

_____ 4.

_____ 5. Occasional or mild inconvenience to family, peers, school or community but still within the normal range; rarely, if ever, enough of a problem to cause any authority (parents, school, law) to intervene strenuously.

_____ 6.

_____ 7. Clear, occasional, mild discomfort to family, peers, school or community; may be one or two instances of intervention by parents or other authorities.

_____ 8.

_____ 9. Frequent mild discomfort to family, peers, school or community; may be several instances of intervention by parents or other authorities.

_____ 10.

_____ 11. Moderate discomfort to family, peers, school or community through physical aggressiveness or destructiveness, legal violations, alcohol or drug involvement, sexual promiscuity, or unusual passivity, apathy, or withdrawal, etc.; likely to have been one or more instances of strenuous interventions by parents or other authorities.

_____ 12.

_____ 13. Severe discomfort or mild danger to family, peers, school or community through behaviors such as those listed in #11 above; likely to have been several instances of strenuous intervention by parents or other authorities.

_____ 14.

_____ 15. Moderate danger to family, peers, school or community; enough to warrant one or two legal or psychiatric incarcerations through behaviors such as those listed in #11 above, at least in part to protect society from the person's actions.

_____ 16.

_____ 17. Severe danger to family, peers, school or community through behaviors such as those listed in #11 above; enough to warrant several brief, or one or two lengthy legal or psychiatric incarcerations, at least in part to protect society from the person's actions.

_____ 18.

_____ 19. Profound danger to family, peers, school or community through accomplishment or genuine threat of actions such as homicide, rape, arson, bombing.

V. *School Performance: Level of academic achievement in relation to actual ability level; rate on the basis of the current semester's performance level.*

_____ 1. Superior level of school performance in relationship to intelligence or ability level; performs above measured IQ or ability level; "overachiever."

_____ 2.

_____ 3. Average level of school performance for IQ or ability level; performs at measured IQ or ability level.

_____ 4.

_____ 5. Level of school performance seems somewhat below ability level, but not extreme enough to be clear underachievement.

_____ 6.

_____ 7. Mild underachievement in one or two courses; that is, person may have one or two courses in which he or she is performing one or two letter grades below his ability level.

_____ 8.

_____ 9. Mild underachievement in most or all courses; that is, person is functioning one or two letter grades below ability level in most or all courses.

_____ 10.

_____ 11. Moderate school underachievement; assuming average or above average intelligence, person is failing one or two core courses.

_____ 12.

_____ 13. Moderate school underachievement; assuming average or above average intelligence, person is failing three core courses.

_____ 14.

_____ 15. Severe school underachievement; assuming average or above average intelligence, person is failing all core courses.

_____ 16.

_____ 17. Severe school underachievement; assuming average or above average intelligence, person is failing all courses.

_____ 18.

_____ 19. Profound school underachievement; person is totally unable to function in the area of academic achievement at this time; or person is out of school at this time.

VI. *Interests: Breadth and depth of interests.*

_____ 1. Unusual range and depth of productive interests.

_____ 2.

_____ 3. Average breadth and depth of interests.

_____ 4.

_____ 5. Some slight restriction in breadth *or* depth of interests.

_____ 6.

_____ 7. Mild but clearly greater than normal restriction in breadth *or* depth of interests; enough restriction to be noted by parents, peers, or teachers.

_____ 8.

_____ 9. Mild but clearly greater than normal restriction in breadth *and* depth of interests; enough restriction to be noted by parents, peers, or teachers.

_____ 10.

_____ 11. Enough restriction in breadth *or* depth of interests to stimulate clear reaction by parents or teachers; interests may not only be restricted but may also tend to be in unrealistic or pathological topics more than healthy ones; for example, person may be interested in activities in the clear absence of relevant skills (grossly unattractive girl wanting to be a teenage fashion model; brain-damaged boy interested in flying airplanes) or may focus on drugs, violence, or self-mutilation more than productive hobbies, athletics, academics, or other positive activities.

_____ 12.

_____ 13. Enough restriction in breadth *and* depth of interests to stimulate clear reaction by parents or teachers; interests may not only be restricted, but may also tend to be in unrealistic or pathological topics more than healthy ones; for example, person may be interested in activities in the clear absence of relevant skills (grossly unattractive girl wanting to be teenage fashion model; brain-damaged boy interested in flying airplanes) or may focus on drugs, violence, or self-mutilation more than productive hobbies, athletics, academics, or other positive activities.

_____ 14.

_____ 15. No genuine interests can be noted; person seems uninterested in anything.

_____ 16.

_____ 17. Of the interests that can be noted, all are clearly bizarre, or severely pathological.

_____ 18.

_____ 19. The only interests that can be noted are lethally destructive (e.g., murder, suicide).

VII. *Intimacy of Relationships: Qualities of interpersonal warmth, intimacy, genuineness, closeness; need to distort perceptions of significant others; stereotypy of relationship style.*

_____ 1. Able to form unusually warm, intimate, undistorted and flexible relationships with a variety of persons.

_____ 2.

_____ 3. Average ability to relate; has several close, meaningful relationships.

_____ 4.

_____ 5. Slight, but definite distance from, or dependency on, significant others; has several close, meaningful relationships at present.

_____ 6.

_____ 7. Mild stereotypy in relationship style; some restriction in choices of relationship objects to persons who fit limited neurotic needs, but still has several close, meaningful and largely non-neurotic relationships.

_____ 8.

_____ 9. Mild stereotypy in relationship style, restriction in choices of relationship objects to persons who fit limited neurotic needs so that no more than one or two can be considered primarily non-neurotic.

_____ 10.

_____ 11. Noticeable lack of genuinely close, warm, intimate relationships; clear distortions in perceptions of others; moderate stereotypy in relationship style, but still has one or two somewhat non-neurotic relationships.

_____ 12.

_____ 13. Noticeable lack of genuinely close, warm, intimate relationships; clear distortions in perceptions of others; moderate stereotypy in relationship style, with all meaningful relationships being dominated by neurotic elements.

_____ 14.

_____ 15. Severe stereotypy, restrictedness, or distortion in the several relationships noted.

_____ 16.

_____ 17. Only one or two clear relationships can be found and these are severely distorted, stereotyped and/or pathological.

_____ 18.

_____ 19. The only relationship that can be noted is profoundly pathological; or the person appears to have no meaningful relationships of any kind at this time.

VIII. *Maturity of Object Relationships: The direction and nature of the person's most meaningful relationship ties.*

_____ 1. Primary relationships are with relatively healthy peers and are quite lasting and stable.

_____ 2.

_____ 3. Primary relationships are with peers of variable psychological health and are of variable duration and stability.

_____ 4.

_____ 5. Primary relationships are with peers of variable psychological health and tend to be relatively brief or stormy.

_____ 6.

_____ 7. Primary relationships seem more or less evenly split between peers and parents (or parent surrogates).

_____ 8.

_____ 9. Primary relationships are with parents (or parent surrogates); the relationships may contain elements of unrealistic idealization.

_____ 10.

_____ 11. Primary relationships are with parents (or parent surrogates); the

relationships may contain distorted elements of hostility and re-
belliousness.

_____ 12.

_____ 13. Extreme tenuousness or apparent absence of significant relationships with peers, parents, or parent surrogates; may relate to animals or inanimate objects; may be shy, lonely, withdrawn or isolated and may, in addition, be grandiose, narcissistic and fragile.

_____ 14.

_____ 15. Clear absence of significant relationships to people, animals, or
inanimate objects; is shy, lonely, withdrawn, or isolated and, in
addition, is grandiose, narcissistic and fragile.

_____ 16.

_____ 17. Any relationships noted are clearly regressed and psychotic and
characterized by primitive identification and ego diffusion; interpersonal affect noted is likely to be extremely aggressive and/or
clinging.

_____ 18.

_____ 19. Any relationships noted are clearly regressed and psychotic and
characterized by primitive identification and ego diffusion; interpersonal affect noted (if any) is likely to be silly, infantile, in-
coherent.

IX. *Insight: The degree to which the person's perception of his/her disturbances corresponds to realistic assessment made by others; acceptance of inner
responsibility; rate on the basis of the person's full conscious awareness,
whether or not he/she will verbally acknowledge awareness of you.*

_____ 1. The person has an unusually deep level of functional understanding of the connections between his/her past experiences, current
feelings, and ongoing behaviors, and typically accepts full personal responsibility for his/her behaviors.

_____ 2.

_____ 3. The person has an average, healthy level of functional understanding of the connections between his/her past experiences,
current feelings, and ongoing behaviors and typically accepts full
responsibility for his/her behaviors.

_____ 4.

_____ 5. The person has a slightly below average, but still basically
healthy, level of functional understanding of the connections between his/her past experiences, current feelings, and ongoing behaviors and usually accepts full responsibility for his/her behaviors.

_____ 6.

_____ 7. Many (but not all) significant areas of disturbance are recognized and the person is usually aware of crucial connections between past experiences, current feelings and behaviors; inner responsibility for behavior is usually accepted and insights are often used to modify behaviors.

_____ 8.

_____ 9. Many (but not all) significant areas of disturbance are recognized, and the person is usually aware of at least some connections between past experiences, current feelings and behaviors; inner responsibility for behavior is usually accepted and insights are often used to modify behaviors.

_____ 10.

_____ 11. Some significant areas of disturbance are recognized, and the person is sometimes aware of the crucial connections between past experiences, current feelings and behaviors; inner responsibility for behavior is sometimes accepted and insights are sometimes used to modify behaviors.

_____ 12.

_____ 13. Some significant areas of disturbance are recognized and the person is sometimes aware of at least some connections between past experiences, current feelings, and behaviors; inner responsibility for behavior is sometimes accepted and insights are sometimes used to modify behaviors.

_____ 14.

_____ 15. Few significant areas of disturbance are recognized, and the person rarely is aware of the crucial connections between past experiences, current feelings, and behaviors; inner responsibility rarely is accepted; instead, there is a heavy reliance on rationalization or minimization; insights rarely are used to modify behaviors.

_____ 16.

_____ 17. Few (if any) significant areas of disturbance are recognized; and the person is rarely (if ever) aware of any connections between past experiences, current feelings, and behaviors; inner responsibility is rarely accepted; instead, there is heavy reliance on projection of blame; insights are rarely used to modify behaviors.

_____ 18.

_____ 19. No significant areas of disturbance are recognized and the person never seems aware of any connections between past experiences, current feelings and behaviors; there is no acceptance of inner responsibility, with blanket denial and gross distortion of the primary means of avoiding responsibility.

X. *Motivation: The amount of goal-directed energy the person can expend toward realistic self-exploration and productive personality change.*

_____ 1. Unusually strongly motivated toward personally and socially productive goals, and very effective in combining realistic goal selection, self-analysis, consistent high energy output, and persistent productive response to frustration.

_____ 2.

_____ 3. Strongly motivated toward personally and socially productive goals and very effective in combining realistic goal selection, self-analysis, consistent high energy output and persistent productive response to frustration.

_____ 4.

_____ 5. Slightly below average but still basically healthy amount of motivation toward personally and socially productive goals, and usually effective in combining realistic goal selection, self-analysis, consistent high energy output and persistent productive response to frustration.

_____ 6.

_____ 7. Clear occasional mild impairment in motivation; may be due to passivity, inability to persevere when frustrated, unwillingness to endure discomfort, inability to risk exposure with therapist and others, or overly restricted goals such as superficial symptom relief, magical "cure," or change in persons other than self.

_____ 8.

_____ 9. Clear continuous mild impairment; may be for reasons similar to those in #7 above.

_____ 10.

_____ 11. Continuous mild impairment in motivation with occasional periods of moderate impairment; may be for reasons similar to those in #7 above but with heavier stress on desire for superficial (or effortless) symptom relief, magical "cures" or changes in persons other than self.

_____ 12.

_____ 13. Continuous moderate impairment in motivation; reasons similar to those in #7 above but with heavier stress on desire for superficial (and effortless) symptom relief, magical "cures," or changes in persons other than self.

_____ 14.

_____ 15. Occasional severe impairment in motivation with chronic mild to moderate impairment; some desire for personal change but only if it does not involve any appreciable energy, frustration, anxiety, depression or risk; tends to persistently demand magic "cure" or change by others rather than self.

_____ 16.

_____ 17. Continuous severe impairment in motivation; may refuse to participate in any treatment in absence of magical changes in others; may perceive treatment as a means of coercing significant people to change their "noxious" manner of dealing with him (or her).

_____ 18.

_____ 19. No apparent motivation to change anything concerning self, significant others, or the environment; person may or may not suffer, have secondary gain, or possess insight, but in any case, person cannot or will not expend any energy in involvement in treatment at any level.

"Liking" Scale

Please rate how strongly you like or dislike this person. Do not add this number into the total psychopathology score!!!

_____ 1. I like this person extremely well.

_____ 2.

_____ 3. I like this person moderately well

_____ 4.

_____ 5. I like this person fairly well.

_____ 6.

_____ 7. I feel neutral or dislike this person mildly.

_____ 8.

_____ 9. I dislike this person moderately.

_____ 10.

_____ 11. I dislike this person extremely.

APPENDIX B

Onset of Symptomatology Scale

I. Psychological Trauma (Age: Birth to Six)
   0. No trauma evident.
   1. —
   2. Somewhat disturbed parenting; must relate to specifics, such as clear, moderate-to-severe neurosis in a parent; clear, mild-to-moderate personality disorder in a parent; clear, mild-to-moderate overcloseness to one parent, with a lack of closeness to the other; six to 12 months' separation from a parent; chronic, mild-to-moderate depression in a parent; or otherwise mildly disturbed family system.
   3. —
   4. Markedly disturbed parenting; must relate to specifics, such as severe personality disorder, clear alcoholism, or psychosis in a parent; severe depression in a parent; loss of a parent through death, desertion, or divorce; severely disturbed family system.

II. Physical Trauma (Age: Birth to Six)
   0. No unusually serious illness, defect, or injury.
   1. Mild physical difficulty in excess of "typical" childhood illness or injury. An example might be premature birth without clear organic damage, or an early history of allergies.
   2. Moderate physical difficulty in excess of "typical" childhood illness or injury. Examples might be diabetes, asthma, convulsions, chronic sickliness, concussion, ulcers, or major surgery.
   3. Severe physical difficulty in excess of "typical" childhood illness or

injury. Examples might be acutely life-threatening defect, illness or injury; includes problems similar to those in level 2, but acutely life-threatening; or strongly suspected minimal brain dysfunction syndrome.

4. Profound physical difficulty in excess of "typical" childhood illness or injury. Examples might be chronic life-threatening defects, illness, or injury; includes problems similar to level 2, but chronically life-threatening; or clear minimal brain dysfunction syndrome.

III. Behavior Control (Age: Birth to Six)

0. Normal management of impulses or feelings.

1. "Overcontrolled"; shy, inhibited, withdrawn, "slow to warm up" child.

2. "Hard to control"; somewhat impulsive, high-tempered, overly aggressive, acting-out child.

3. "Very hard to control"; moderate-to-severe impulsivity, hyperactivity, or belligerently aggressive, acting-out child.

4. Bizarre child; psychotic-like losses of control, or very peculiar impulse and need gratification management (rocking, severe headbanging, posturing, self-biting, peculiar gestures, etc.).

IV. Academic Progress (Age: Six to Hospital Admission)

0. No failures through twelfth grade; or may have "underachieved" from seventh to twelfth grades.

1. One or more F's from tenth through twelfth; or may have "underachieved" from first to sixth grades.

2. One or more F's from seventh through ninth grades.

3. One or more grade failures from fourth through sixth grades.

4. One or more grade failures from first through third grades.

V. Peer Relationships (Age: Six to Hospital Admission)

0. No particular problems establishing or maintaining friendships.

1. Loss of previous ability to establish or maintain friendships at age 13–16, due to withdrawal, unpleasantness, or change in choice of friends to markedly immature peers.

2. Many years' trouble relating to peers—shy, withdrawn, a "loner"; few, if any, close friends ever.

3. Many years' trouble relating to peers—controlling, aggressive, "obnoxious"; or no really close, warm relationships but may have one or few (generally male) peers as antisocial companions.

4. Peer scapegoat; generally functions as the butt of peers' hostility.

VI. Passivity-Aggressiveness Deviance (Age: Six to Hospital Admission)

0. Normal assertiveness.

1. —

2. Clearly passive and/or aggressive physically or verbally.

3. —

4. Profoundly passive and/or physically aggressive to a life-threatening degree.

VII. Symptom Duration (Age: Birth to Hospitalization)

0. No moderate-to-severe neurotic, personality disorder, or psychotic symptoms noted for more than six months prior to admission.

1. Moderate-to-severe neurotic, personality disorder, or psychotic symptoms noted six to 12 months prior to admission.

2. Moderate-to-severe neurotic, personality disorder, or psychotic symptoms noted one to three years prior to admission.

3. Moderate-to-severe neurotic, personality disorder, or psychotic symptoms noted four to six years prior to admission.

4. Moderate-to-severe neurotic, personality disorder, or psychotic symptoms noted more than six years prior to admission.

APPENDIX C

Beavers-Timberlawn
Family Evaluation
Scale

BEAVERS-TIMBERLAWN FAMILY EVALUATION SCALE

Rater.................................

Date.................................

Family Name.................................

Segment.................................

Instructions: The following scales were designed to assess the family functioning on continua representing interactional aspects of being a family. Therefore, it is important that you consider the entire range of each scale when you make your ratings. Please try to *respond on the basis of the videotape data alone*, scoring according to what you see and hear, rather than what you imagine might occur elsewhere.

I. *Structure of the Family*

A. Overt Power: Based on the entire tape, check the term that best describes your general impression of the overt power relationships of this family.

1	1.5	2	2.5	3	3.5	4	4.5	5
Chaos		Marked dominance		Moderate dominance		Led		Egalitarian
Leaderless; no one has enough power to structure the interaction.		Control is close to absolute. No negotiation; dominance and submission are the rule.		Control is close to absolute. Some negotiation, but dominance and submission are the rule.		Tendency toward dominance and submission, but most of the interaction is through respectful negotiation.		Leadership is shared between parents, changing with the nature of the interaction.

194

B. Parental Coalitions: Check the terms that best describe the relationship structure in this family.

1	1.5	2	2.5	3	3.5	4	4.5	5
Parent-child coalition				Weak parental coalition				Strong parental coalition

C. Closeness

1	1.5	2	2.5	3	3.5	4	4.5	5
Amorphous, vague and indistinct boundaries among members				Isolation, distancing				Closeness, with distinct boundaries among members

II. *Mythology:* Every family has a mythology; that is, a concept of how it functions as a group. Rate the degree to which this family's mythology seems congruent with reality.

1	1.5	2	2.5	3	3.5	4	4.5	5
Very congruent		Mostly congruent				Somewhat incongruent		Very incongruent

III. *Goal-Directed Negotiation:* Rate this family's overall efficiency in negotiating problem solutions.

1	1.5	2	2.5	3	3.5	4	4.5	5
Extremely efficient		Good				Poor		Extremely inefficient

IV. *Autonomy*

A. Clarity of Expression: Rate this family as to the clarity of disclosure of feelings and thoughts. This is not a rating of the intensity or variety of feelings, but rather of clarity of individual thoughts and feelings.

1	1.5	2	2.5	3	3.5	4	4.5	5
Very clear				Somewhat vague and hidden				Hardly anyone is ever clear

B. Responsibility: Rate the degree to which the family members take responsibility for their own past, present, and future actions.

1	1.5	2	2.5	3	3.5	4	4.5	5
Members regularly are able to voice responsibility for individual actions				Members sometimes voice responsibility for individual actions, but tactics also include sometimes blaming others, speaking in 3rd person or plural				Members rarely, if ever, voice responsibility for individual actions

C. Invasiveness: Rate the degree to which the members speak for one another, or make "mind reading" statements.

1	1.5	2	2.5	3	3.5	4	4.5	5
Many invasions				Occasional invasions				No evidence of invasions

D. Permeability: Rate the degree to which members are open, receptive and permeable to the statements of other family members.

1	1.5	2	2.5	3	3.5	4	4.5	5
Very open		Moderately open				Members frequently unreceptive		Members unreceptive

197

V. *Family Affect*

A. Range of Feelings: Rate the degree to which this family system is characterized by a wide range expression of feelings.

1	1.5	2	2.5	3	3.5	4	4.5	5
Direct expression of a wide range of feelings		Direct expression of many feelings despite some difficulty			Obvious restriction in the expressions of some feelings	Although some feelings are expressed, there is masking of most feelings		Little or no expression of feelings

B. Mood and Tone: Rate the feeling tone of this family's interaction.

1	1.5	2	2.5	3	3.5	4	4.5	5
Usually warm, affectionate, humorous and optimistic		Polite, without impressive warmth or affection; or frequently hostile with times of pleasure		Overtly hostile		Depressed		Cynical, hopeless and pessimistic

C. Unresolvable Conflict: Rate the degree of seemingly unresolvable conflict.

1	1.5	2	2.5	3	3.5	4	4.5	5
Severe conflict, with severe impairment of group functioning		Definite conflict, with moderate impairment of group functioning		Definite conflict, with slight impairment of group functioning		Some evidence of unresolvable conflict, without impairment of group functioning		Little, or no unresolvable conflict

D. Empathy: Rate the degree of sensitivity to, and understanding of, each other's feelings within this family.

1	1.5	2	2.5	3	3.5	4	4.5	5
Consistent empathic responsiveness		For the most part, an empathic responsiveness with one another, despite obvious resistance		Attempted empathic involvement, but failed to maintain it		Absence of any empathic responsiveness		Grossly inappropriate responses to feelings

VI. *Global Health-Pathology Scale: Circle the number of the point on the following scale that best describes this family's health or pathology.*

10	9	8	7	6	5	4	3	2	1
Most Pathological									Healthiest

199

APPENDIX D

Main Study Follow-up Interview Schedule

Name of Subject _____ Name of Ex-Patient _____

Relationship of Subject to Ex-Patient _____

Discharge Date _____ Date of Interview _____

Time from Discharge to Follow-Up Interview _____

Location of Interview _____

Instructions to Interviewer:

Explain the purpose of the follow-up interview.

Emphasize your desire to learn more about how the ex-patient has personally experienced his or her life since discharge, and also explain our use of de-identified feedback for improvement of our treatment programs.

Present the consent form with a full explanation, sign the consent form, and obtain the subject's signature.

Request permission to audiotape the interview, with assurance that sensitive or intimate portions of the interview will be deleted from the tape at the subject's request.

I. *Subject's Narrative Account*

Begin the interview with an open-ended question, something like, "Mr. Smith, you left Timberlawn 2½ years ago. Fill me in on where you've been, what you've been doing, and how things have been for you over that period of time."

Or, if interviewing a parent or spouse, begin with a statement such as "Mrs. Smith, your husband left Timberlawn 2½ years ago. Fill me in on what he has done and how things have gone for him in that period of time." Take detailed notes in the space below, and on the back of the page.

200

II. *Friends and Social Life*

Ask for a description of the ex-patient's friendship and peer relationships, details of social life, and quality of relationships reported. Obtain information concerning the general number of male and female friends, an estimate of closeness of the relationships, and some idea of how the ex-patient organizes social leisure time.

Obtain information about intimate or romantic relationships, including dating patterns, approximate dates of living together, engagement, marriage, separation, or divorce.

Request information about pregnancies, abortions, miscarriages, or children resulting from intimate relationships.

Take detailed notes in the space below.

III. *Relationships with Parents*

Ask an open-ended question about the ex-patient's current relationship with parents. Obtain information about post-discharge living arrangements (with parents, apartment, with spouse, and so forth).

Inquire specifically about the presence of conflicts between the ex-patient and each parent. Inquire whether the current relationship with parents is similar to, or different from that which existed at the time of hospitalization, and inquire about reasons for differences that are reported.

Assess the degrees of affection and respect felt for each parent.

IV. *Occupational Activities*

Inquire specifically about schools attended, academic level of function, degrees, diplomas, or other certification obtained, with approximate dates of attendance.

Inquire specifically about jobs held, nature of vocational activity, approximate dates of employment, and reasons for leaving each job reported. Inquire about anticipated future educational and vocational activities.

For ex-patients not enrolled in school or involved in paid employment (such as full-time homemakers, for example), inquire specifically about daily activities to get a picture of the means of structuring time. Inquire about special interests, hobbies, and talents.

V. *Miscellaneous*

A. Inquire about serious physical illnesses or accidents since hospital discharge.

B. Ask about patterns of usage of alcohol, marijuana, prescribed and non-prescribed drugs. Ask if the ex-patient has had any personal, family, physical, or legal troubles related to alcohol, marijuana, or drug usage since discharge.

C. Inquire about other possible problems with legal authorities.

D. Ask for information pertaining to psychiatric rehospitalization since discharge, obtaining the name of hospital, approximate dates of hospitalization, precipitating factors, and outcome of treatment.

E. Inquire about outpatient, individual, group, marital, or family therapy, or other counseling contacts since discharge. Obtain names of therapists, approximate dates of treatment, an explanation for reasons of termination, and a description of treatment results.

VI. *Description of Inpatient Treatment at Timberlawn*

A. Ask about feelings about the hospital treatment program in which the ex-patient was involved while at Timberlawn.

B. Ask for a listing and explanation of everything recalled that seemed *helpful* during hospitalization.

C. Ask for a listing and explanation of everything that seemed *non-helpful* or *harmful* during inpatient treatment.

If this interview is being conducted with the ex-patient, indicate your desire to contact a spouse or parent for a collaborative interview. Emphasize the value of the collaborative interview, and assure the ex-patient of total confidentiality of all information in the current interview. Obtain names, telephone numbers, and addresses with which to contact the spouse or parent for the collaborative interview.

VII. *Mental Status*

Note any significant factors or special problems encountered in scheduling the interview.

Record detailed notes concerning the subject's appearance and style in the interview.

This *Follow-Up Interview Schedule* is not meant to be a detailed or sufficient guide for untrained or inexperienced interviewers. On the contrary, this *Schedule* is intended to serve as a general outline and format for organized note-taking for trained and skilled mental health professional interviewers.

We would appreciate being contacted by anyone using this *Schedule*.

John T. Gossett, Ph.D.
Timberlawn Psychiatric Research
   Foundation
2750 Grove Hill Road
P.O. Box 270789
Dallas, Texas 75227
214/388-0451

APPENDIX E

Medication
Dose Levels

Medication	Mg/day	
	Low**	High
Antipsychotic Dose Levels*		
Thorazine	≤ 999	≥ 1000
Mellaril	≤ 799	≥ 800
Quide	≤ 99	≥ 100
Stelazine	≤ 49	≥ 50
Navane	≤ 49	≥ 50
Haldol	≤ 24	≥ 25
Tricyclic Antidepressant Dose Levels*		
Elavil	≤ 299	≥ 300
Sedative Dose Levels*		
Chloral Hydrate	≤ 999	≥ 1000
Placidyl	≤ 999	≥ 1000

(continued)

| Sodium Butisol | ≤ 99 | ≥ 100 |
| Dalmane | ≤ 29 | ≥ 30 |

Minor Tranquilizer Dose Levels*

| Librium | ≤ 79 | ≥ 80 |
| Valium | ≤ 39 | ≥ 40 |

*If two or more medications are used concurrently, use milligram equivalents to find combined dose level.

**Medication dose levels determined by Gregory Dimijian, M.D., and Larry E. Tripp, M.D.

Index

205

Suicide, 60, 65, 79, 82, 92, 139, 144, 161, 179, 180
Symptoms:
  chronicity of and long-term outcome, 91–97
  duration of, measurement of, 93, 95–97, 103, 192
  onset of:
    gradualness of, 18, 20
    intensity of, 92
    multivariate analysis of, 126–31
    in pilot study, 38–39, 43–45, 47
    process, 17–22, 25, 38–39, 43–45
    rate of, 92
    reactive, 17–22, 25, 38–39, 43–45, 47, 139
    and sexuality, 92
  rate of change early in hospitalization, 92

Tantrums, 19
Telephone contact, 9, 41, 55, 58, 73, 167
Termination of treatment, type of in pilot study, 40, 43–45
Tests, psychological, 9, 12
Thomas, A., 40, 49n.
Thorazine, dosages of, 203
Ticks, 19
Timberlawn Adolescent Service, 33, 48, 53, 61

Timberlawn Psychiatric Research Foundation, 55
Tranquilizers. *See also* Sedatives
  major and minor, 107–109
  dosages of, 203–204
Tricyclic antidepressants, dosages of, 203. *See also* Antidepressant drugs
Tripp, L. E., 108n., 204n.
Truancy, 57
Turner, D. R., 40n.

Unconscious defense, 9
Underachievement. *See* Academic performance
Unitization of hospital facilities, 28
Utilization Review, 135, 162

Vaillant, G. E., vii–viii
Valium, dosages of, 204
Values, family, 151
Vandalism, 18, 19, 54, 57
Vocational training, 149. *See also* Occupational functioning

Warren, W., 21, 31n.
Wechsler Adult Intelligence Scale, 70
Wechsler Intelligence Scale for Children, 70
Work adjustment, 41
Working-through, 149